Dominik F.L. Freund

Measuring Sales Efficiency in the Pharmaceutical Industry

Dominik F.L. Freund

Measuring Sales Efficiency in the Pharmaceutical Industry

New Horizons in Sales Controlling

Südwestdeutscher Verlag für Hochschulschriften

Impressum/Imprint (nur für Deutschland/ only for Germany)
Bibliografische Information der Deutschen Nationalbibliothek: Die Deutsche Nationalbibliothek
verzeichnet diese Publikation in der Deutschen Nationalbibliografie; detaillierte bibliografische
Daten sind im Internet über http://dnb.d-nb.de abrufbar.
Alle in diesem Buch genannten Marken und Produktnamen unterliegen warenzeichen-, marken-
oder patentrechtlichem Schutz bzw. sind Warenzeichen oder eingetragene Warenzeichen der
jeweiligen Inhaber. Die Wiedergabe von Marken, Produktnamen, Gebrauchsnamen,
Handelsnamen, Warenbezeichnungen u.s.w. in diesem Werk berechtigt auch ohne besondere
Kennzeichnung nicht zu der Annahme, dass solche Namen im Sinne der Warenzeichen- und
Markenschutzgesetzgebung als frei zu betrachten wären und daher von jedermann benutzt
werden dürften.

Verlag: Südwestdeutscher Verlag für Hochschulschriften Aktiengesellschaft & Co. KG
Dudweiler Landstr. 99, 66123 Saarbrücken, Deutschland
Telefon +49 681 37 20 271-1, Telefax +49 681 37 20 271-0, Email: info@svh-verlag.de
Zugl.: Wien, WU, Diss., 2008

Herstellung in Deutschland:
Schaltungsdienst Lange o.H.G., Berlin
Books on Demand GmbH, Norderstedt
Reha GmbH, Saarbrücken
Amazon Distribution GmbH, Leipzig
ISBN: 978-3-8381-0982-4

Imprint (only for USA, GB)
Bibliographic information published by the Deutsche Nationalbibliothek: The Deutsche
Nationalbibliothek lists this publication in the Deutsche Nationalbibliografie; detailed
bibliographic data are available in the Internet at http://dnb.d-nb.de.
Any brand names and product names mentioned in this book are subject to trademark, brand or
patent protection and are trademarks or registered trademarks of their respective holders. The
use of brand names, product names, common names, trade names, product descriptions etc.
even without a particular marking in this works is in no way to be construed to mean that such
names may be regarded as unrestricted in respect of trademark and brand protection legislation
and could thus be used by anyone.

Publisher:
Südwestdeutscher Verlag für Hochschulschriften Aktiengesellschaft & Co. KG
Dudweiler Landstr. 99, 66123 Saarbrücken, Germany
Phone +49 681 37 20 271-1, Fax +49 681 37 20 271-0, Email: info@svh-verlag.de

Copyright © 2009 by the author and Südwestdeutscher Verlag für Hochschulschriften
Aktiengesellschaft & Co. KG and licensors
All rights reserved. Saarbrücken 2009

Printed in the U.S.A.
Printed in the U.K. by (see last page)
ISBN: 978-3-8381-0982-4

Measuring sales efficiency in the pharmaceutical industry

Table of contents:

Table of contents i
List of figures iii
List of tables vi
Glossary ix
Abstract x
1   Introduction 1
   1.1   Problems and objectives 1
   1.2   Proceeding 4
2   Theoretical bases of efficiency analysis and description of the methods used 5
   2.1   Literature overview 5
   2.2   Terms and definitions of productivity and efficiency 11
      2.2.1   Relationship between productivity and efficiency 11
      2.2.2   Technical, allocative, scale and overall efficiency 13
   2.3   Efficiency analyses regarding frontier functions 17
   2.4   Measuring concepts for evaluating efficiency 18
      2.4.1   Model with constant returns to scale (CRS) 20
      2.4.2   Model with variable returns to scale (VRS) 25
      2.4.3   The slack based measurement model 28
      2.4.4   The super efficiency model 31
      2.4.5   The Malmquist Productivity Index 33
   2.5   Concepts used: Management cockpit and efficiency gap 39
      2.5.1   The management cockpit 40
      2.5.2   The efficiency gap 44
   2.6   Software used 47
3   Data, definitions and characteristics of the pharmaceutical sales process 49
   3.1   Data and Definitions 51
      3.1.1   Sales Process Productivity (SPP) Definitions 52
      3.1.2   Output Definitions 54

	3.1.3	Reinterpreting the share of market (SOM)	55
	3.1.4	Combining inputs and outputs into one data sheet	56
3.2		Current sales representative benchmarking system	57
4		Empirical efficiency analyses	60
4.1		Results of the CCR model	62
	4.1.1	CCR DEA Version 1 (F, CCD, CCP, F/T - Q, CI)	63
	4.1.2	Summary of the CCR DEA model	70
4.2		Results of the BCC model	79
	4.2.1	DEA setting with four inputs and two outputs (F, CCD, CCP, F/T - Q, CI)	79
	4.2.2	Summary of the BCC DEA model	86
4.3		Results of the inter-temporal, non orientated SBM model with VRS	93
	4.3.1	SBM Model Version 1 (F, CCD, CCP, F/T, Q, CI)	97
	4.3.2	SBM Model Version 2 (F, CCD, F/T, - Q, CI)	113
	4.3.3	SBM Model Version 3 (F, CCD, CCP, F/T - SOM)	125
	4.3.4	SBM Model Version 4 (F, CCD, CCP, F/T - TR)	136
	4.3.5	SBM Model Version 5 (F, CCD, F/T, TR)	147
	4.3.6	Summary of the SBM DEA model	159
5		Summary and Conclusion	172
6		References	188
7		Appendix	193
7.1		Appendix A	193
7.2		Appendix B	196
	7.2.1	Appendix B1 (NO-SBM-V model, Version: F, CCD, CCP, F/T – Q, CI)	197
	7.2.2	Appendix B2 (CCR-Model, Version: F, CCD, CCP, F/T – Q, CI)	207
	7.2.3	Appendix B3 (BCC-Model, Version: F, CCD, CCP, F/T – Q, CI)	211
	7.2.4	Appendix B4 (input orientated SBM model with CRS)	215

List of figures

Figure 2.1-1: Difference between effectiveness and efficiency 7
Figure 2.1-2: Approaches to Salesperson Performance Evaluation 8
Figure 2.2.2-1: Technical, Allocative and Overall Efficiency 13
Figure 2.4.1-1: Input orientated CCR example 22
Figure 2.4.2-1: CRS and VRS – showing the difference graphically 26
Figure 2.4.4-1: Input orientated ranking of efficient units – basic idea 32
Figure 2.4.5-1: Catch up process and frontier shift from period 1 to 2 34
Figure 2.4.5-2: Productivity change and relative efficiency over time 38
Figure 2.5.1-1: Example for a management cockpit in DEA 41
Figure 2.5.2-1: Example of an efficiency gap illustration 45
Figure 3-1: Insulin market growth from 1999 to 2006 50
Figure 3-2: Deterioration of the share of market (SOM) from the q1 2004 to q4 2006 ... 50
Figure 4.1.1-1: Illustration of the Efficiency Gap and of the three efficiency groups 63
Figure 4.1.1-2: KPI-Cockpit for SR 4 67
Figure 4.1.1-3: KPI-Cockpit for SR 28 68
Figure 4.1.1-4: KPI-Cockpit for SR 42 69
Figure 4.1.2-1: Efficiency gap comparison of the different CCR DEA versions 70
Figure 4.1.2-2: Difference in BCC and CCR output projection 78
Figure 4.2.1-1: The efficiency gap for the BCC model version 1 79
Figure 4.2.1-2: KPI Cockpit for SR4 84
Figure 4.2.1-3: KPI Cockpit for SR28 84
Figure 4.2.1-4: KPI Cockpit for SR42 85
Figure 4.2.2-1: Summary of the efficiency gap for the BCC DEA versions 86
Figure 4.3.1-1: Illustration of the Efficiency Gap and of the three efficiency groups 97
Figure 4.3.1-2: Development of average input and output values over time 104
Figure 4.3.1-3: KPI-Cockpit for SR 4 107
Figure 4.3.1-4: Decomposition of the MPI and presentation of the development of relative efficiency 108
Figure 4.3.1-5: KPI-Cockpit for SR 28 110

Figure 4.3.1-6: Decomposition of the MPI and presentation of the development of relative efficiency 110
Figure 4.3.1-7: KPI-Cockpit for SR 42 111
Figure 4.3.1-8: Decomposition of the MPI and presentation of the development of relative efficiency 112
Figure 4.3.2-1: Illustration of the Efficiency Gap and of the three efficiency groups 113
Figure 4.3.2-2: Development of average input and output values over time 117
Figure 4.3.2-3: KPI-Cockpit for SR 4 (F, CCD, F/T – Q,CI) 119
Figure 4.3.2-4: Decomposition of the MPI and the efficiency development of SR4 120
Figure 4.3.2-5: KPI-Cockpit for SR 28 (F, CCD, F/T – Q,CI) 121
Figure 4.3.2-6: Decomposition of the MPI and the efficiency development of SR28 ... 122
Figure 4.3.2-7: KPI-Cockpit for SR 28 (F, CCD, F/T – Q, CI) 123
Figure 4.3.2-8: Decomposition of the MPI and the efficiency development of SR42 ... 124
Figure 4.3.3-1: Illustration of the Efficiency Gap and of the three efficiency groups 125
Figure 4.3.3-2: Development of average input and output values over time 129
Figure 4.3.3-3: KPI-Cockpit for SR 4 (F, CCD, CCP, F/T – SOM) 131
Figure 4.3.3-4: Decomposition of the MPI and the efficiency development of SR4 132
Figure 4.3.3-5: KPI-Cockpit for SR 28 (F, CCD, CCP, F/T – SOM) 133
Figure 4.3.3-6: Decomposition of the MPI and the efficiency development of SR28 ... 134
Figure 4.3.3-7: KPI-Cockpit for SR 42 (F, CCD, CCP, F/T – SOM) 134
Figure 4.3.3-8: Decomposition of the MPI and the efficiency development of SR42 ... 135
Figure 4.3.4-1: Illustration of the Efficiency Gap and of the three efficiency groups 136
Figure 4.3.4-2: Development of average input and output values over time 140
Figure 4.3.4-3: KPI-Cockpit for SR 4 (F, CCD, CCP, F/T – TR) 142
Figure 4.3.4-4: Decomposition of the MPI and the efficiency development of SR4 143
Figure 4.3.4-5: KPI-Cockpit for SR 28 (F, CCD, CCP, F/T – TR) 144
Figure 4.3.4-6: Decomposition of the MPI and the efficiency development of SR28 ... 144
Figure 4.3.4-7: KPI-Cockpit for SR 42 (F, CCD, CCP, F/T – SOM) 145
Figure 4.3.4-8: Decomposition of the MPI and the efficiency development of SR42 ... 146
Figure 4.3.5-1: Illustration of the Efficiency Gap and of the three efficiency groups 147
Figure 4.3.5-2: Development of average input and output values over time 151
Figure 4.3.5-3: KPI-Cockpit for SR 4 (F, CCD, CCP, F/T – TR) 153
Figure 4.3.5-4: Decomposition of the MPI and the efficiency development of SR4 154

Figure 4.3.5-5: KPI-Cockpit for SR 28 (F, CCD, F/T – TR) 155
Figure 4.3.5-6: Decomposition of the Malmquistindex and development
of relative efficiency 156
Figure 4.3.5-7: KPI-Cockpit for SR 42 (F, CCD, CCP, F/T – SOM) 157
Figure 4.3.5-8: Decomposition of the Malmquistindex and efficiency
development for SR42 158
Figure 4.3.6-1: Comparison of the different efficiency gaps 159
Figure 4.3.6-2: Efficiency developments over time for the different DEA settings 160
Figure 4.3.6-3: Development of the MPI for the different DEA versions for SR4 164
Figure 4.3.6-4: Development of the MPI for the different DEA versions for SR28 167
Figure 4.3.6-5: Development of the MPI for the different DEA versions for SR28 169
Figure 5-1: Increase in efficiency for SR28 by deleting the inefficiencies in the specific
dimensions 177
Figure 7.2-1: Production possibility set P and frontiers 194
Figure 7.2-2: Production possibility set P´ and frontiers 194

List of tables

Table 3.1.1-1: Example for calculating the average monthly call capacity of a quarter .. 53
Table 3.1.2-1: Excerpt of output data for a sales rep 54
Table 3.1.4-1: Excerpt of the data sheet for the DEA analysis 57
Table 3.1.4-2: Different DEA versions analysed within this thesis 57
Table 3.2-1: Evaluation system for realizations in different dimension 58
Table 3.2-2: Evaluation table of ten exemplary sales reps 59
Table 4.1.1-1: Differences between the efficiency groups 64
Table 4.1.1-2: Optimal projection – opportunity cost of inefficiency 66
Table 4.1.2-1: Summarized results for SR4 71
Table 4.1.2-2: Summarized results for SR28 72
Table 4.1.2-3: Summarized results for SR42 73
Table 4.1.2-4 Frequency of efficient benchmarks 74
Table 4.1.2-5: Impact factors of the efficient sales reps in the different CCR version 75
Table 4.1.2-6: Overall insulin and market share increases in case of efficient operation 76
Table 4.1.2-7: Maximum projection and maximum value achieved 77
Table 4.2.1-1: Results of the BCC and CCR model 80
Table 4.2.1-2: Differences between the efficiency groups 81
Table 4.2.1-3: Optimal input and output projection for the BCC DEA model version 1 .. 83
Table 4.2.2-1: Summary of SR4 for the different BCC DEA versions 87
Table 4.2.2-2: Summary of SR28 for the different BCC DEA versions 88
Table 4.2.2-3: Summary of SR42 for the different BCC DEA versions 89
Table 4.2.2-4: Frequencies of efficient sales reps 90
Table 4.2.2-5: Impact factors of the efficient sales reps as benchmark for the sample .. 91
Table 4.2.2-6: Optimal output projections for the five BCC DEA versions 91
Table 4.3.1-1: Comparison of average efficiency scores 98
Table 4.3.1-2: Relationship between average efficiency scores and multipliers 101
Table 4.3.1-3: Average virtual worth of the input or output category 102
Table 4.3.1-4: Comparison of current and optimal target values 102
Table 4.3.1-5: Average productivity development described by the average MPI 105
Table 4.3.1-6: Development of Ø efficiency 105

Table 4.3.2-1: Comparison of average efficiency scores 113
Table 4.3.2-2: Relationship between average efficiency scores and multipliers 115
Table 4.3.2-3: Average virtual worth of the input or output category 116
Table 4.3.2-4: Comparison of current and optimal target values 116
Table 4.3.2-5: Average productivity development described by the overall MPI 118
Table 4.3.2-6: Development of Ø efficiency 118
Table 4.3.3-1: Comparison of average efficiency scores 126
Table 4.3.3-2: Sources of efficiency for the different groups 127
Table 4.3.3-3: Average virtual worth of the input or output category 128
Table 4.3.3-4: Comparison of current and optimal target values 128
Table 4.3.3-5: Average productivity development described by the overall MPI 130
Table 4.3.3-6: Development of Ø efficiency 130
Table 4.3.4-1: Comparison of average efficiency scores 137
Table 4.3.4-2: Results of the Mann Whitney U Test to identify reasons for efficieny ... 138
Table 4.3.4-3: Average virtual worth of the input or output category 139
Table 4.3.4-4: Comparison of current and optimal target values 139
Table 4.3.4-5: Average productivity development described by the overall MPI 141
Table 4.3.4-6 Development of Ø efficiency 141
Table 4.3.5-1: Comparison of average efficiency scores 148
Table 4.3.5-2: Results of the Mann Whitney U Test to identify sources of efficiency ... 149
Table 4.3.5-3: Average virtual worth of the input or output category 150
Table 4.3.5-4: Comparison of current and optimal target values 150
Table 4.3.5-5: Development of the MPI over time 152
Table 4.3.5-6: Development of Ø efficiency 152
Table 4.3.6-1: Significance of differences in the efficiency scores 161
Table 4.3.6-2: Evidence for the positive effect of Q on efficiency 161
Table 4.3.6-3: The difference of Q/SOM between the quartiles disappears 162
Table 4.3.6-4: Summary of SR4 163
Table 4.3.6-5: Summary of SR 28 166
Table 4.3.6-6: Summary of SR 42 168
Table 4.3.6-7: Frequencies of efficient sales reps 170
Table 4.3.6-8: Cumulated weights of the benchmark partners 171
Table 4.3.6-9: Insulin increases: absolute and in terms of market share 171

Table 5-1: Sensitivity of (super) efficiency scores to changes in the DEA models 175
Table 5-2: Characteristic determinants of the different DEA versions 179
Table 5-3: Characteristic differences between groups regarding efficiency 180
Table 7.2-1: Super Efficiency Datasheet – Input orientated 193
Table 7.3-1: Data sheet for the fourth quarter 2006. 196
Table 7.3-2: Average values of the dimensions over the relevant time interval 196
Table 7.3.1-1: Decomposition of inefficiency for the different sales reps 197
Table 7.3.1-2: The table on the left displays the slacks for the sample 198
Table 7.3.1-3: Individual input and output virtual weights for the sample 199
Table 7.3.1-4: Weighted data set, i.e. the virtual weights times the data 200
Table 7.3.1-5: Individual benchmark partners for inefficient sales reps 201
Table 7.3.1-6: Status quo value for q4 2006 and the optimized target values 202
Table 7.3.1-7: Displays the efficiency scores over time from q1 2004 to q4 2006 203
Table 7.3.1-8: The catch up process of the individual sales reps 204
Table 7.3.1-9: The frontier shift of the individual sales reps 205
Table 7.3.1-10: The Malmquist Productivity Index of the individual sales reps 206
Table 7.3.2-1: Slack values for the CCR model version 1 for each sales reps 207
Table 7.3.2-2: Displays the virtual weights for the CCR model version 1 208
Table 7.3.2-3: Displays the individual benchmark partners for inefficient sales reps ... 209
Table 7.3.2-4: Status quo value for q4 2006 and the optimized target values 210
Table 7.3.3-1: Slack values for the BCC model version 1 for each sales reps 211
Table 7.3.3-2: Virtual weights for the BCC model version 1 212
Table 7.3.3-3: Individual benchmark partners for inefficient sales reps 213
Table 7.3.3-4: The table on the left displays the status quo value for q4 2006 214
Table 7.3.4-1: Data set with big variations in input 1 and input 2. 215
Table 7.3.4-2: Results of the MWU-Test with big variations in input 2. 216
Table 7.3.4-3: Data set with big variations in input 1 and small variations in input 2. .. 217
Table 7.3.4-4: Results of the MWU-Test for with small variations in input 2. 217

Glossary

BCC	DEA model named after Banker, Charnes and Cooper with variable returns to scale
CCD	Input: Call Capacity to Doctors
CCP	Input: Call Capacity to Pharmacies
CCR	DEA model named after Charnes, Cooper and Rhodes with constant returns to scale
CI	Output: Competition Index
CRS	Constant returns to scale
CU	Catch Up Process
DMU	Decision Making Unit
e	e denotes a row vector in which all elements are equal to 1.
F	Input: Frequency
FS	Frontier Shift
F/T	Input: Relation of fixed doctors to total doctors
MPI	Malmquist Productivity Index
NO-SBM-V	Non orientated, slack based measurement model with variable returns to scale
Q	Output: Quantity of insuling sold in
SOM	Output: Share of market
$\sum_{j=1}^{n} \lambda_j$	indicates the sum of $\lambda_1 + \lambda_2 + ... + \lambda_n$.
$\sum_{j=1; j \neq k}^{n} \lambda_j$	indicates the sum with λ_k omitted: $\lambda_1 + ... + \lambda_{k-1} + \lambda_{k+1} ... + \lambda_n$.
SR X	Sales representative X
TR	Output: Target realization
VRS	Variable returns to scale
x, y, λ	Small letters in bold face denote vectors.

Abstract

A recurring, but unresolved issue in sales force research is the choice of the sales force evaluation method. In this thesis the author applies Data Envelopment Analysis (DEA) to the topic of sales force evaluation. Due to the fact that DEA applications in sales force evaluations are on a nascent stage the existing literature is extended to an inter-temporal DEA approach with a productivity index, to assess performance evaluation of salesmen over time. The DEA model used to assess the sales force is called the slack based measurement model (SBM). The calculated efficiency scores of the SBM model are decomposable and, therefore, those input and output dimension, which contribute the worst to the efficiency scores calculated, are identified. The main advantage of the SBM model is that it does not distinguish between weak and strong efficient units. Moreover the analysis identifies criteria for choosing an optimal DEA version in sales. In addition, the concept of super-efficiency is applied for ranking efficient sales representatives. Using the shadow prices the author tries to identify more and less important input and output variables for a DEA analysis in sales. The assessment of individuals in sales is based on several input and output factors. In current sales force assessments multiple input and output factors result in subjective benchmarks, due to subjectively chosen weights. To overcome this situation, DEA is empirically applied to a sales force of a well known pharmaceutical company to incorporate all relevant key performance indicators into one single, objective efficiency measure for all individuals in the sample.

Last but not least, the results of this analysis determine an alternative way to existing methods of sales controlling.

Keywords:

Data Envelopment Analysis, non orientated slack based measurement model, Malmquist Productivity Index, super efficiency, shadow prices, decomposition of efficiency, choice of variables

1 Introduction

Data Envelopment Analysis (DEA) measures the relative efficiency of multiple "Decision Making Units" (DMU) when multiple inputs and outputs are present. This general set up is applicable for many different topics one of which is sales force evaluation. In this thesis DEA is applied to the insulin sales force of a well known pharmaceutical company to develop a new and more detailed method for sales force evaluation. The existing DEA literature is extended by new methods, which allow a more in-depth analysis.

1.1 Problems and objectives

The sales market for pharmaceutical products is characterized by strong competition (see Schumacher and Reiß 2006). As companies are seeking for increasing market shares they expect and face growing sales activities. These expectations are based on different factors:

- In view of greater complexity and shorter innovation cycles for new drugs it gets more and more important to allow for highly qualified and intensive communication efforts between **p**harmaceutical **c**ompanies (**PC**) and their customers.
- In addition, the steadily decreasing "time to market" of new products gives birth to higher demands regarding sales representatives of pc´s.
- Despite the fact of rising direct mail sellings the physician itself will remain the central contact person for pc´s.

This type of communication between pcs and customers demands a large field sales force, today as well as in future. Consequently, the expenditures for sales and marketing are as high as 25% to 30% of turnover. At the same time the distribution of innovative drugs requires high qualifications of sales representatives: a large portion of sales representatives have got an academic background. The forecast for the future development of sales and marketing is ambivalent: On the one hand pc´s will be forced to reduce costs stemming from turnover decreases due to patent expiration, which will hit field sales force as well. Due to declining product differentiation and shorter exclusivity periods for drugs on the other hand dense market coverage and *sophisticated sales channel control systems* will be indispensable: highly qualified sales representatives consult prescribing specialist, like oncologists for cancer and neurologists for MS, Parkinson and psychological illnesses or endocrinologists for diabetics.

Considering the points mentioned above sales managers have to be evaluated in a sophisticated manner guaranteeing high sales performance. This is where efficiency measurement plays an important role. For a pc it is important to know about the efficiency of its sales force to detect failures, shortcomings and improvement potential.

Which sales units are efficient performers and which are inefficient ones and why?

The first question arising at this stage will be: which efficiency measure shall a company use to assess sales personnel?
Several different methods are worth thinking of. In general a division into non-parametric and parametric methods for efficiency measurement is conceivable. In addition simpler evaluation systems (i.e. summing up weighted scores) are in common use across companies.
In this dissertation the focus is on the non-parametrical Data Envelopment Analysis and the results of the DEA study will be discussed in the light of the currently used "best praxis" method of the company.

Worldwide the non-parametrical Data Envelopment Analyses has developed into an increasingly important efficiency measurement tool (see Taveres (2002)). DEA reveals it self to be a powerful efficiency measurement tool not only because it can easily handle multiple inputs and outputs, but also because it is capable of processing qualitative and quantitative inputs and outputs with different units.
With regards to these two main advantages, DEA has gained enormous popularity among researchers and managers.
But still – there remains a lot of research to be done. One field of research remaining is within sales controlling, especially in the pharmaceutical industry. In addition, this study is one of the first applying the Malmquist Productivity Index (MPI) and its decomposition based on a non-radial, non-orientated slack based measurement model. Cooper, Seiford and Tone (2007)

mention, that empirical application using this promising method are on a nascent stage and, thus, worth for further analysis. In addition the resulting efficiency scores will be decomposed.

Questions of interest are:

1. Is DEA in general applicable to this subject?
2. Which DEA version and model[1] (static/inter-temporal) is the most suitable?
3. What are the differences in comparison to currently prevailing performance measurement methods?

In the following sections these methodical questions for efficiency measurement will be highlighted and viewed from several different directions.

An empirical example is examined using DEA to answer these questions relating to efficiency measurement methods. The author will take a closer look at the functioning of sales controlling of one of the world biggest pharmaceutical companies. The current methods for controlling sales representatives will be described and analysed and compared to the DEA approach.

Besides the methodological questions, questions of economic concern will be answered. Such as:

1. How do sales units differ with regard to economic success and efficiency?
2. Which connection exists between efficiency and the input and output dimensions?
3. How big are the potential savings of production factors for the different sales units and how large are potential turn over increases?

---

[1] Version: input and output setting; Model: CCR, BCC or SBM (for details see chapter 2.4)

1.2 Proceeding

This dissertation is divided into 7 chapters. The introduction provides basic information on the pharmaceutical industry concerning the topic of sales.

Chapter 2 present's a literature overview concerning articles and papers written about efficiency measurement in sales controlling and different models for measuring efficiency. The chapter deals with theoretical backgrounds of all efficiency measurement tools which will be used in this thesis. Furthermore concepts are presented how to communicate DEA results to the management in a comprehensible way.

In chapter 3 the specific characteristics of the analysed insulin sales force are presented together with the market situation in the country of interest. The data and definitions used within this thesis are outlined and the evaluation system which is currently applied by the company will be presented.

Chapter 4 is divided into several subchapters and each subchapter presents the results of a different DEA versions (the different input and output mixes) and model (variable returns to scale or constant returns to scale, non-orientated or output orientated). Several different input and output mixes will be evaluated in connection with inter-temporal aspects which highlight the development of productivity over time. In addition the results are compared with each other and the different performance indicators will be highlighted. The conclusions drawn in chapter 4 focus on the results of the *specific* DEA model and version applied. Therefore recommendations for sales rep improvements will be given according to the specific DEA results. For easy comparisons of results each subchapter of the analysis is structured in the same way. The aim is to find implications of changing DEA settings regarding the whole sample and to identify the impact of these implications on an individual level.

Chapter 5 extends the summary and conclusion to a more general view. The different versions will be compared considering their impact on the efficiency score and then an optimal DEA version and model is tried to be identified. Furthermore the currently used evaluation system is compared to the DEA model.

Chapter 6 lists the references used for this thesis and chapter 7 contains the appendices[2].

---

[2] To avoid overstretching the volume of this book, the appendix B only presents the complete data for input and output version 1 calculated with the CCR, BCC and SBM model. All other data can be requested via email (dominik.freund@gmx.de).

2 Theoretical bases of efficiency analysis and description of the methods used

Chapter 2 begins with a literature overview which presents the field of research and finally highlights open research questions. The terms productivity and efficiency will be defined. In addition the different efficiency measurement methods are presented in detail.

2.1 Literature overview

Strong competition and rising pressure on sales men demand fair and precise benchmarking tools. Fair benchmarking tools resolve into a transparent perception of personal sales performance evaluation which increases satisfaction within the sales force. In the end transparent benchmarking increases overall sales performance and therefore is of crucial importance for every company. Hence, salesperson performance evaluation is a frequent matter in sales force research.

Measuring sales force performance reaches back several decades. In the seventies, sales performance measurement started to broaden. Sales performance was assessed either by *qualitative* or *quantitative* measures. Sales managers and researchers were constantly searching for the relationship between personal characteristics and personal traits and the successful salesman. Mostly a single measure of sales success was used to describe a multidimensional problem and bivariate statistical techniques were applied to multivariate relationships (see Lamont et al., 1977).

Qualitative measures such as territory management, customer relation, knowledge and experience can be structured through the use of behaviour anchored rating scales (BARS) which were first applied to the topic of sales performance measurement by Cocanougher and Ivancevich 1978. BARS is a procedure that attempts to provide data indicating how performance can be improved. Cocanougher and Ivancevich mention that it is assumed that management can, through the utilization of the BARS approach, determine what behaviours are associated with achieving desired results.

Quantitative measures include output measures like sales or quota attainment, input measures such as number of calls and time utilization or include ratio measures like expense ratios, account development and service ratios (see Churchill et al. 1990).

General speaking outputs focus on employee results and inputs draw attention to the actions or efforts of the salesperson and how those are undertaken.
In addition researchers distinguish controllable variables which can be influenced through managerial decisions on the one side from non controllable variables like territory workload (see Cravens, LaForge, Pickett and Young 1993) and market potential on the other side.

A further way of assessing sales is utilizing group performance evaluations. Group performance measurement can be divided into three main groups (see Eichel and Bender 1984). (A)The comparative method which compares employees with each other in the form of rankings, distributions or paired comparisons etc. (B) A different type of group performance measurements are outcome based evaluations which measure and compare the results of salespersons efforts. (C) Absolute appraisal methods on the other hand include behaviours as inputs of a group.

Each of the measures mentioned above refers to either *objectivity* or *subjectivity* and to either *efficiency* or *effectiveness*.
The difference between efficiency and effectiveness is that effectiveness focuses on the contribution of salespersons to generate outcomes like total quantity sold or market share. Efficiency on the other hand highlights the process which is utilized to reach managerial predetermined sales volumes or market shares.

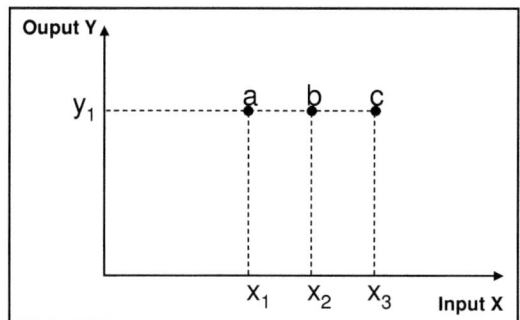

Figure 2.2.1-1: Difference between effectiveness and efficiency

Figure 2.2.1-1 highlights this fact. Points a, b and c represent three decision making units (DMU). Each DMU produces the same amount of output y_1. Henceforth all three are effective in producing the output y_1. But only DMU "a" is the most efficient. This is because it produces y_1 with the least input amount x_1 in comparison to the larger input amounts of DMU "b" and DMU "c".

In the literature of sales performance measurement the focus seems to be on effectiveness rather than efficiency.

In today's competitive environments dominated by cost cutting programmes and production maximisation the focus of scientific sales performance measurement methods should concentrate on both effectiveness and efficiency.

Boles et. al. (1995) integrate pre '95 performance conceptualizations into four groups based on their use of input and output measures. Because the pre'95 literature on sales scarcely accounts for concepts of effectiveness **and** efficiency these are not represented in the first four groups. Therefore a fifth group is added which includes the concepts of effectiveness and efficiency (see Figure 2.2.1-2).

In this fifth group the concept of Data Envelopment Analysis (DEA) is added. Under this approach a salespersons performance is compared to the best performer within the evaluated sample. The best performer is the one who maximizes outputs with respect to inputs. The measures incorporated into the DEA approach can be subjective and/or objective.

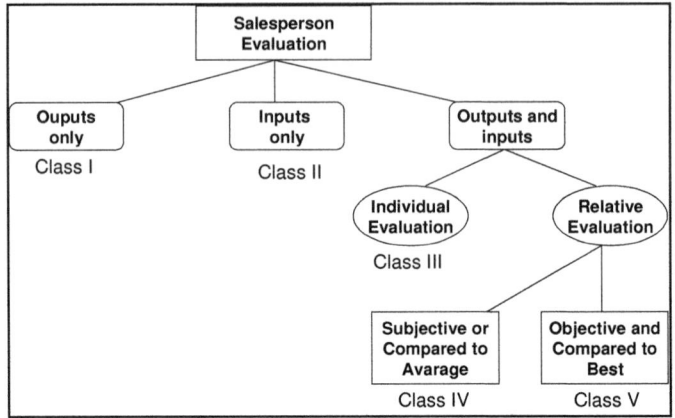

Figure 2.2.1-2: Approaches to Salesperson Performance Evaluation;
Source: Boles et al. (1995)

Boles et al. (1995) are the first to apply the DEA method to evaluate sales performance. Therefore the author of this proposal proposes to present an overview of the main pre´1995 literature following Boles and from 1995 onward to concentrate on DEA approaches for sales evaluation presented after 1995.

Before post 1995 DEA literature is presented, examples of the different "salesperson evaluation classes" (see Figure 2.2.1-2) are given.

Class I literature focuses on results as the criteria of evaluation. Both objective (e.g., sales volume) and subjective (e.g., achieving sales objectives) can be used. Bagozzi (1978) presents a model designed to explain the performance, job satisfaction and other behavioural outcomes experienced by salespeople. For example he estimates results (sales) as function of subjective measures such as self-esteem, verbal intelligence, job related tension and objective measures such as workload and territory potential. The independently variable self-esteem which is used to estimate sales is itself a dependent variable to another regression problem. Hastings et al. (1988) focus on output and measures the sales increase invoked through different incentive methods.

Class I evaluation methods do not benchmark a salesperson directly to another, but the results can be used to rank salespeople for purposes of comparison.

The general advantage of output orientated methods is that they highlight a firm's base line performance. A disadvantage may be that these methods underlie a narrow view due to their reliance on output measures only. Effectiveness may be measured but not efficiency.

Class II literature concentrates on inputs as measure for sales performance. These input measures could be objective measures such as sales calls made or subjective measures such as salesmanship skills. These measures are than compared against performance goals. For example Sager and Varadarajan (1990) measure performance using an 87 item sales representative performance appraisal form related to in-store activities, relationship with supervisors and sales presentation. Week et al. (1990) analyse the time spent with potential customers by salesmen. The study investigates whether time spent calling on established accounts and potential accounts affects different measures of sales force performance.
In addition it is examined whether these relationships vary across career stages.
Input focused approaches according to Class II therefore may be helpful for firms that use performance evaluation to discover an individual's trainings and development needs.

The next class takes into account inputs and outputs and hence relates the individual sales process and its different characteristics to the achieved sales results. For example Lamont (1977) tries to reveal the relationship between personality variables and personal characteristics and measures of sales performance by using objective and subjective measures. In doing this he relates several different variables for sales performance (e.g., sales quota, new business conversion, managerial ratings (e.g., technical competence, territory management, salesmanship skills etc.)), for personality (e.g., dominance, endurance, social recognition etc.) and for personal characteristics (e.g., age, height, weight etc.) to another. An additional example is the article of Avila, Fern and Mann (1988). They relate the input measures sales behaviour and goal achievement to sales managers´ overall performance assessment and try to reveal the relationship between sales behaviours and the degree to which salespeople meet sales goals and how managers arrive at overall performance assessments.
Class III and the other two classes of evaluation methods have in common that they do not explicitly compare a salesperson with his or her peers, but can be rank-ordered for purpose of comparison.

The fourth class of literature goes one step further. In this class the evaluation methods define a standard in order to explicitly compare salespeople to their peers. This aim can be achieved in several ways. One way is to compare one individual with other salespeople through supervisory or self-reported ratings (e.g. see Kohli 1989). Another way is using regression based methods which relate inputs and outputs of
salespersons and which compare the outcomes with the mean rating (see Lucas, Weinberg, and Clowes 1975). Both supervisory and regression based methods have crucial shortcomings. Supervisory methods lack on the fact that they are mainly based on subjective standards and the problem with regression based methods is, by definition, that they only use average performance as the bases for relative evaluations.

Finally class V is meant to incorporate objective and compared to best methods.
Boles et al. (1995) introduce Data Envelopment Analysis (DEA) in sales performance evaluation to meet this task.
DEA is a relative performance measurement method which incorporates multiple inputs and outputs simultaneously. These inputs and outputs can be subjective and objective. DEA views performance as a relative efficiency measure and benchmarks each sales individual against the best of the analysed sample.
For the analysis of sales personnel Boles takes four inputs and three outputs into consideration using a DEA model with constant returns to scale. The output measures used were percentage of sales quota attained, a three-item supervisor evaluation of overall salesperson performance and sales volume in US $. The inputs measures were sales experience (number of months the salesperson had been in a sales position with the firm), salary, management ratio (ratio of managers in the office to salespeople assigned to that office) and territory potential.
All input and output variables are treated as controllable variables in the evaluation approach of Boles. This fact is critical when it comes to territory potential which can not be influenced by management like the other variables.
In addition Boles applies a static DEA to evaluate sales performance and does not take into account inter temporal effects.

Pilling et al. (1998) addresses the problem of different territory potential in sales person's evaluation within a DEA framework. He utilizes territory data of members of a national association of apparel manufactures. The data included input dimensions like total market demand for the industry in question (apparel industry), average sales per account, and growth rate of market demand for that industry. Territory characteristics were accounted for as inputs and then individual salesperson's relative performance efficiencies were computed taking into account the two outputs actual and perceptual sales volume. Actual measures report actual sales volume. Perceptual measures report the individual salesman's perception of sales volume and include perceptions relative to other salespeople. The DEA was run in a standard CCR (assuming constant returns to scale) setup treating all inputs and outputs as controllable ones.

Though DEA has been applied to numerous sales activities (Thomas et al. 1998, Donthu and Yoo 1998, Luo 2003, de Mateo et al. 2006) it has not been extensively applied to the case of individual salesmen (Boles et al. 1995, Pilling et al. 1999), performance evaluation.

2.2 Terms and definitions of productivity and efficiency

In this sub-section productivity and efficiency are examined as a basis for further presentations of efficiency measurement methods. Included is a break down of the term efficiency into different types of efficiencies that will be important for understanding.

2.2.1 Relationship between productivity and efficiency

Central to evaluating a sales representative or a so called "decision making unit" (DMU), is to measure its productivity and to compare the resulting productivity with the productivity outcomes of other DMU´s within a given period.
In general productivity can be written as:

$$\frac{Output}{Input}$$

This general definition can be applied to numerous questions. An important distinction has to be set between partial factor productivity (PFP) and total factor productivity (TFP). Taking into consideration PFP a focus is laid upon a partial relationship which takes particular inputs and outputs into account. These are elements of a production process which uses multiple inputs and outputs. TFP, for instance, accounts for all inputs and outputs used within a production process. In this dissertation the TFP is of major interest because the DEA can include all relevant inputs and outputs and, therefore, provides a holistic view of the production process. Basically, productivity expresses the relationship between outputs and inputs for a specific DMU at a certain point in time.

Efficiency, though describes the unused potential of productivity or, to state it differently otherwise, the diversion between the observed productivity from the optimal possible productivity.

Therefore, measuring and analysing efficiency is of major importance in order to show potential of productivity increases. Both efficiency and productivity of a DMU are determined through the production technology used and from uncontrollable external factors.

T.C. Koopmans (1951) was the first to formally define efficiency in the context of production economics.

Two definitions of efficiency can be quoted:

> Definition 1: *(Pareto-Koopmans Definition of Efficiency) The performance of a DMU is efficient if and only if it is not possible to improve any input or output without worsening any other input or output.*

From the first definition the following one can be derived:

> Definition 2: *(Definition of Inefficiency) the performance of a DMU is inefficient if and only if it is possible to improve some input or output without worsening some other input and output.*

Keeping these two definitions in mind it is possible to look at the task of measuring efficiency from two different ways. The first possibility of analysing efficiency is an output orientated one. The underlying question here is to which extent outputs can be increased using the given inputs. If outputs of a DMU cannot be increased without increasing its inputs, the considered DMU must be efficient.

The second option of analysing efficiency is an input orientated one. The underlying question in this case is to which extent inputs can be reduced keeping current output levels constant. If inputs of a DMU can not be reduced further without reducing outputs at the same time, it must be efficient.

Frankly speaking, in the output case the search is for a maximum expansion of outputs for given inputs and in the input case for a minimum endowment with inputs to produce a given output. In addition Tone (2001) developed a method which optimizes both the inputs and outputs simultaneously which will be discussed in chapter 2.4.3.

2.2.2 Technical, allocative, scale and overall efficiency

Before introducing different efficiency analysing methods, it is important to distinguish between the diverse efficiency terms which are often used to describe different states of efficiency.

In contrast to overall efficiency, which includes technical and allocative efficiency, technical efficiency focuses on the purely "technological" aspects of production. It does not take into account prices or other valuing information.

In addition to technical efficiency, a production process works allocative efficient if it takes optimal price or other optimal valuing information into account. Figure 2.2.2-1 presents the details.

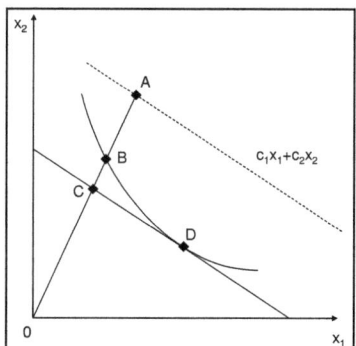

Figure 2.2.2-1: Technical, Allocative and Overall Efficiency

The curved line in Figure 2.2.2-1 represents a segment of an isoquant that stands for all input combinations (x_1, x_2) that are needed to optimally produce the same amount of a single output. All points along the isoquant are technical efficient. Hence the isoquant stands for an efficiency frontier.

Each point which lies above the isoquant along the ray from the origin to point A represents the same amount of output produced with the same input ration but with different amounts of input. All other points which lie above the isoquant but not on the ray represent the same amount of output but they are, in fact produced with a different input mix than the ones on the ray. The budget lines $c_1x_1+c_2x_2$ are represented through the parallel broken and solid line, the former representing total costs of k_0 and the latter of k_1. The dotted line depicts higher costs and the solid line lower costs, $c_1x_1+c_2x_2=k_1 < c_1x_1+c_2x_2=k_0$.

Thus point A is technical and allocative inefficient because it produces the same amount of the single output that is produced along the isoquant at higher costs.
According to Farrell (1957), it is possible to measure the so called *radial efficiency*. The measure can be presented in the following ratio which relates the distance from the origin to the different points, here:

$$0 \leq \frac{\overline{OB}}{\overline{OA}} \leq 1$$

The result is the measure of technical efficiency that is from now on labelled θ.

When taking allocative efficiency into account prices have to be considered. The broken line intersecting with point A is associated with production costs of k_1. Nevertheless, these costs can be reduced by shifting the broken line parallel downward until it intersects with point D, where total costs amount to k_0. The difference between k_1 and k_0 shows the extent to which costs can be reduced. Point D is the allocation with the minimal possible production costs for an output amount represented on the isoquant. A further reduction of cost would lead to a decrease in outputs. Point C is not feasible as a production point, but it can be used for evaluating the allocative efficiency of point B:

$$0 \leq \frac{\overline{OC}}{\overline{OB}} \leq 1$$

The allocative efficiency shows which extent the technical efficient point B fails to achieve minimal costs. This inefficiency is a result of the failure to not make the substitutions involved from A to D along the efficiency frontier.

"Overall efficiency" is represented by

$$0 \leq \frac{\overline{OC}}{\overline{OA}} \leq 1$$

This measure represents the amount to which the original point A falls short of achieving minimal costs.

As can be easily demonstrated through

$$\frac{\overline{OB}}{\overline{OA}} * \frac{\overline{OC}}{\overline{OB}} = \frac{\overline{OC}}{\overline{OA}},$$

the technical efficiency times the allocative efficiency is equal to the overall efficiency.

Technical efficiency can be decomposed into the so called pure technical efficiency and scale efficiency.
The relationship can be depicted as (see Cooper, Seiford and Tone 2006)

technical efficiency = pure technical efficiency * scale efficiency

If investigating the source of technical inefficiency it is important to know if the inefficiency is mainly because the DMU is badly operated or due to disadvantageous conditions in which the DMU is functioning under. These disadvantageous conditions have their source in different returns to scale that are induced through dissimilar DMU size. The DMU operating at most productive scale size (MPSS) has constant returns to scale and DMU's producing more output than at the MPSS imply decreasing returns to scale and units producing beneath the MPSS imply increasing returns to scale. These differences in scale size lead to inefficiencies.
At this stage this is enough information. The author refers to chapter 2.4.2 for a deeper analysis of scale efficiency.

For now it should be sufficient to mention that the scale efficiency is calculated by relating a model with constant returns to scale to a model with variable returns to scale. The result has to be smaller than or equal to unity and is called scale efficiency. The technical efficiency divided by the scale efficiency results in the pure technical efficiency. As mentioned above the pure technical efficiency spots the inefficiency occurring caused by a weak operation.

2.3 Efficiency analyses regarding frontier functions

Different methods can be used to measure the technical efficiency of a DMU. In this dissertation the technical efficiency of DMU's is measured with frontier models. Taking all the observations into account, a production function is produced and this function represents the efficiency frontier.
Ideally, all of these frontier functions should lead to a single efficiency measure for all the different DMU's incorporating variables with different scaling and with different measurement units.

In the literature, the approaches for efficiency measurement are divided into parametric and non-parametric methods. In addition, the literature distinguishes between stochastic and deterministic approaches.
The difference between parametric and non-parametric approaches is that a parametric method assumes some sort of production function *a priori* and estimates the parameters with statistical methods and empirical data. Advantageous in comparison to non-parametric methods is the fact that the parametric methods can account for stochastic variations in the data set and, therefore, is not so sensitive to outliers.
In contrast to parametric methods, non-parametric methods take advantage of linear-programming to find a tight envelope for the empirical data set. Crucial is the fact that the non-parametric method does not assume a production function *a priori* and is sensitive to outliers.

In addition, frontier measurement methods can either be deterministic or stochastic. Deterministic methods use the maximum possible output to determine the production function. Stochastic approaches take a random disturbance term into account, so that the production frontier is not solely determined by the production factors but is also determined by random fluctuations.

In the literature, the methods mentioned above have their supporters and critics. It is not clear which one is the best. For efficiency measurement the deterministic DEA and the parametric stochastic frontier analysis (SFA) have evolved as the ones most frequently used. However, in this thesis efficiency evaluation with DEA will be assessed.

2.4 Measuring concepts for evaluating efficiency

In the following subsection, the different measuring concepts for evaluating efficiency will be presented. The section starts with the basic DEA models and carries on presenting some more advanced DEA application which will be useful for sales evaluation. In addition the "Malmquist-Productivity-Index" as an instrument to evaluate productivity changes of the whole sample and of single sales representatives will be discussed.
The subsection closes with a short presentation of the software used in this work.

The main advantage of non parametric efficiency measurement is that no functional form of a production function has to be assumed *a priori*. Instead, an envelopment function is laid around the empirical data with the help of linear optimization. Due to the fact that non parametric deterministic methods such as DEA do not account for random errors in the data, they are very sensitive to outliers. Hence, it is decisive to check for the quality of the data before starting an efficiency measurement.

Theoretical bases of Data Envelopment Analysis (DEA)

DEA has been recognized as an analytical research instrument and a practical decision support tool. DEA transforms multi dimensional input- and output measures into a single efficiency measure. An important fact about DEA is that it calculates objective weights for each input and output of every DMU under consideration through linear optimization. As a result, optimal weights for inputs and outputs are calculated for every DMU in relation to all DMU´s under consideration. Because of its objectivity, the DEA results can be widely accepted by both management and evaluated DMU´s.
In addition, the efficiency of a DMU is always measured in relation to DMU´s which underlie a similar production structure and which, therefore, always are situated closely to oneanother on the production frontier. This, of course, is advantageous for drawing strategic conclusions from the analysis results.

Another positive feature of DEA is the fact that data with non monetary dimensions can be handled as easily as data classified in monetary dimensions. This makes DEA very flexible in its use.

An important fact to mention is the relation between DMU and considered variables. The more variables are chosen, the more DMU´s will be efficient. If the number of DMU´s is relatively small and the number of variables relatively low, then a large amount of DMU´s will lie on the efficiency frontier. In this case, the result of the analysis will be that most of the DMU´s are efficient. This fact, of course, alters every analysis in the sense of making it worthless if the relationship between DMU´s and variables is unfavourable.

In the literature, the relationship between DMU´s and variables varies but it should be at least 3:1 (Cooper, Seiford and Tone 2006).

In the following subsections, the DEA models taken into account in this thesis will be presented. Firstly a, model with constant returns to scale, than a model with variable returns to scale and finally, the possibility of inter temporal DEA analysis with help of the windows analysis will be presented.

The CCR model evaluates n DMU´s with the input and output matrices $X=(x_{ij}) \in \mathbb{R}^{m \times n}$ and $Y=(y_{rj}) \in \mathbb{R}^{s \times n}$. It is assumed that the data set is positive, i.e. $\mathbf{X}>0$ and $\mathbf{Y}>0$. The production possibility set P is defined as $P = \{(\mathbf{x},\mathbf{y}) | \mathbf{x} \geq \mathbf{X}\lambda,\ \mathbf{y} \leq \mathbf{Y}\lambda,\ \lambda \geq 0\}$ where λ is a nonnegative vector in $\mathbb{R}^n$.

2.4.1 Model with constant returns to scale (CRS)

The basic DEA model was developed by Charnes et al. in 1978 and implied constant returns to scale. In the literature, it is therefore, titled as CRS-model (see Zhu 2002) or after the authors as CCR-model (see Cooper et al. 2007). The model is a so called radial model because it measures the inefficiency of a DMU through its radial distance from the production function frontier.

The basic idea of DEA is to assign one efficiency value to each DMU_j (j=1,...,n). This efficiency value is calculated through the ratio of all weighted outputs y_r (r=1,...,s) and of all weighted inputs x_i (i=1,...,m). The efficiency value for a single DMU can be described by the following formula:

$$\frac{Y}{X} = \frac{\sum_{r=1}^{s} u_r y_r}{\sum_{i=1}^{m} v_i x_i}$$

Inputs and outputs with different dimension are made comparable through the introduction of aggregation weights (v,u). These weights are not estimated *a priori*, they are results of the optimisation process. For each and every DMU the weights are calculated in such a manner that they maximise efficiency values of a DMU in comparison with all other DMU´s. In addition the efficiency values for the DMU´s are restricted to a maximum level of one[3]. If a DMU reaches a level of one it operates efficiently. Furthermore, the weights are restricted to being non negative. The following fractional optimization problem results for DMU_o:

$$\max_{v,u} \theta = \frac{u_1 y_{10} + u_2 y_{20} + ... + u_s y_{so}}{v_1 x_{10} + v_2 x_{20} + ... + v_m x_{mo}} = \frac{\sum_{r=1}^{s} u_r y_{ro}}{\sum_{i=1}^{m} v_i x_{io}}$$

(2-1) subject to

$$\frac{u_1 y_{1j} + ... + u_s y_{sj}}{v_1 x_{1j} + ... + v_m x_{mj}} = \frac{\sum_{r=1}^{s} u_r y_{rj}}{\sum_{i=1}^{m} v_i x_{ij}} \leq 1$$

$$u_s \geq 0$$
$$v_i \geq 0$$

---

[3] A special version of DEA, the Super efficiency model is able to calculate scores greater than one for example to rank efficient units.

The objective is to obtain weights v_i and u_r that maximise the ratio of DMU_o, the DMU being evaluated, so that the efficiency value θ is maximised. θ is a scalar ranging from 0 to 1. V_i and u_r can be defined as shadow prices (or virtual weights) and indicate the usage intensity of an input or output factor in the production process of a DMU. The model (2.1) is a fractional program which can result in an infinite number of solutions. Standardization of the weighted input sum to one transforms (2.1) into a linear optimization problem which has a definite solution:

(2-2) subject to

$$\max_{\mu,v} \theta = \sum_{r=1}^{s} \mu_r y_{ro}$$

$$\sum_{i=1}^{m} v_i x_{io} = 1$$
$$\sum_{r=1}^{s} \mu_r y_{rj} \leq \sum_{i=1}^{m} v_i x_{ij}$$
$$v_i \geq 0$$
$$\mu_r \geq 0$$

The model (2-2) is an **input orientated** CCR-model which can be solved using the simplex algorithm. The outcome of linear program (2-2) is the maximum efficiency value θ for the DMU under evaluation and the respective weights μ, v which are necessary to achieve the maximum efficiency value of θ.

In Figure 2.4.1-1, all DMUs produce the same amount of output. Three DMU's represent the efficiency frontier. DMU 5 is inefficient and DMU 4 is situated on the efficiency frontier but uses an excessive amount of input 1. Therefore, DMU 4 is regarded as weak efficient because it could reduce input 2 without lowering the level of output. DMU 5 is radial inefficient because it can improve efficiency along the ray through the origin by a proportional reduction of its inputs. DMU 4 is mix inefficient because it has to change its input mix to reach the efficiency frontier.

To account for mix inefficiencies as well, a **two stage** optimization problem has to be introduced.

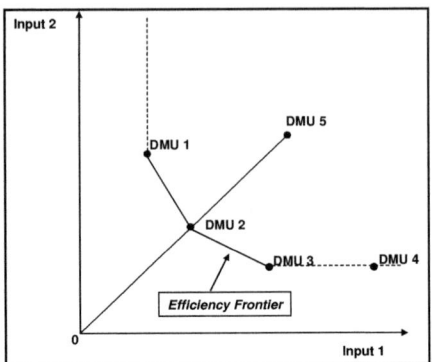

Figure 2.4.1-1: Input orientated CCR example

Considering the duality theorem it is possible to transform (2-2) into a dual model which results in the same efficiency values as (2-2). But it implies different interpretation possibilities. At this **first** stage the efficiency value θ is calculated:

$$\min_{\theta, \lambda} \theta$$

(2-3)   subject to

$$\sum_{j=1}^{n} \lambda_j x_{ij} \leq \theta x_{io}$$
$$\sum_{j=1}^{n} \lambda_j y_{rj} \geq y_{ro}$$
$$\lambda_j \geq 0$$

For DMU 5 in Figure 2.4.1-1, an optimal $\theta^*_{DMU5} \leq 1$ results. (*with stars indicating optimal values*) DMU 2 is the only benchmark partner of DMU 5. This is indicated through $\lambda_{DMU2} = 1$ and $\lambda_j = 0$ ($j \neq DMU2$). Thus, DMU 5 should reduce inputs to the amounts of DMU 2.

Solving equation (2-3) for DMU 4 results in $\theta^*_{DMU4} = 1$ which is the same efficiency score as for DMU´s 1 and 3. As mentioned above, DMU 4 is situated on the efficiency frontier and, after solving (2.3), reaches an efficient status. But, obviously, DMU4 is mix inefficient[4] and can reduce input 1 without reducing input 2 and the produced output amount. An optimization potential which originates from mix inefficiencies is called a *slack value*.

---

[4] Mix inefficiency: in this case: being on the efficiency frontier but with a suboptimal input mix.

Perhaps both input and output slacks exist in model (2-3). After calculating equation (2-3) usually the following situation occurs:

a) $s_i^- = \theta^* x_{io} - \sum_{j=1}^{n} \lambda_j x_{ij}$

b) $s_r^+ = \sum_{j=1}^{n} \lambda_j y_{rj} - y_{ro}$

Where s_i^- indicates an input slack and s_r^+ an output slack. After model (2-3) is solved, in a **second** stage optimization the maximal excess values of s_i^- and s_r^+ are detected by solving the following linear programming model to determine the non-zero slacks:

$$\max \sum_{i=1}^{m} s_i^- + \sum_{r=1}^{s} s_r^+$$

(2-4) subject to

$$\sum_{j=1}^{n} \lambda_j x_{ij} + s_i^- = \theta^* x_{io}$$

$$\sum_{j=1}^{n} \lambda_j y_{rj} - s_r^+ = y_{ro}$$

$$\lambda_j \geq 0$$

A DMU is strong efficient if and only if $\theta^* = 1$ and $s_i^- = s_r^+ = 0$ for all i and r. The first (2-3) and second (2-4) stage optimization can be involved in a single DEA model:

$$\min \theta - \varepsilon \left(\sum_{i=1}^{m} s_i^- + \sum_{r=1}^{s} s_r^+ \right)$$

(2-5) subject to

$$\sum_{j=1}^{n} \lambda_j x_{ij} + s_i^- = \theta^* x_{io}$$

$$\sum_{j=1}^{n} \lambda_j y_{rj} - s_r^+ = y_{ro}$$

$$\lambda_j \geq 0$$

ε is a non-Archimedean number and effectively allows the minimization over θ to pre-empt the optimization involving the slacks, s_i^- and s_r^+. The model (2-5) is the envelopment form of DEA including the slack calculation, and model (2-2) is the multiplier form of DEA. The first (2-5) calculates the efficient values of θ^* of each DMU and indicates the reference or benchmark partners of inefficient DMUs through λ. The latter (2-2) results in the efficiency value θ* of each DMU due to duality as well and calculates the optimal weights or shadow prices v, μ for each DMU which indicate factor usage intensity of the specific inputs and outputs with respect to the objective.

The models above are input orientated. In addition output orientated models exist within the DEA context. To compute an output orientated model the weighted sum of outputs in model (2-1) is standardized to 1. The primal, output orientated CCR-model can than be written as:

(2-6)

$$\min_{\mu,v} \phi = \sum_{i=1}^{m} v_i x_{io}$$

subject to

$$\sum_{r=1}^{s} \mu_r y_{ro} = 1$$
$$\sum_{i=1}^{m} v_i x_{ij} \leq \sum_{r=1}^{s} \mu_r y_{rj}$$
$$v_i \geq 0$$
$$\mu_r \geq 0$$

With $\phi = \frac{1}{\theta}$. The two stage dual formulation of the output orientated model than is:

(2-7)

$$\max \phi - \varepsilon \left(\sum_{i=1}^{m} s_i^- + \sum_{r=1}^{s} s_r^+ \right)$$

subject to

$$\sum_{j=1}^{n} \lambda_j x_{ij} + s_i^- = x_{io}$$
$$\sum_{j=1}^{n} \lambda_j y_{rj} - s_r^+ = \phi^* y_{ro}$$
$$\lambda_j \geq 0$$

Models (2-6) and (2-7) can be interpreted in an analogous way as like the input orientated models. Here, the optimal values of the objective functions indicate to which extend output can be increased, given constant input levels.

A main disadvantage of the models introduced so far is that they assume constant returns of scale. In most cases this assumption does not hold in reality.

2.4.2 Model with variable returns to scale (VRS)

However, in a lot of cases variable returns to scale seem to be the appropriate assumption. To account for variable returns to scale Banker, Cooper and Charnes developed a DEA model, which is called the BCC-model (see Banker et al. 1984).

The assumption of VRS allows for non proportional increases or decreases of outputs when the input values are changed. In addition, the most productive scale size (MPSS) can be determined under which a DMU produces under constant returns to scale. Figure 2.4.2-1 shows both, the CRS efficiency frontier and the frontier under variable returns to scale.

The switch from CRS to VRS influences the whole efficiency frontier. Under CRS only DMU B is efficient. All other DMUs are inefficient. Under variable returns of scale the envelope covers the observations closer and therefore, DMU A, C and D are also efficient. DMU B remains unchanged and hence efficient. Under the assumption of VRS, DMU B continues to exhibit CRS as it is the only DMU which lies on both the VRS and CRS efficiency frontier. Yet, DMU E and F remain inefficient under VRS. But the degree of inefficiency of DMU E and F has decreased due to the fact that they are located closer to VRS efficiency frontier. The changes occurring when switching from CRS to VRS reveal the general tendency, that under VRS more units as under CRS are efficient and that the degree of inefficiency decreases for all evaluated units under VRS compared to the situation under CRS (see Banker et al. 1984)[5].

---

[5] For empirical evidence check the appendix C for the calculations of the BCC and CCR efficiency scores.

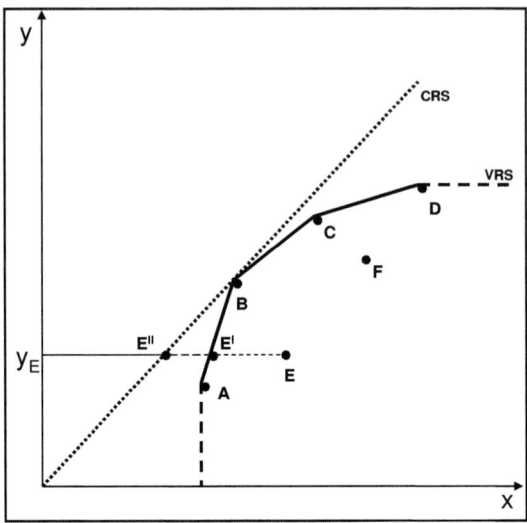

Figure 2.4.2-1: CRS and VRS – showing the difference graphically

Figure 2.4.2-1 sheds light on another interesting fact. It shows the amount of inefficiency experienced by DMU E due to an impropriate scale size indicated by $\overline{E^{II}E^{I}}$. Then the remaining inefficiency $\overline{E^{I}E}$ reveals the inefficiency attributable solely to bad operation which is also named the pure technical inefficiency.

Mathematically the input orientated multiplier VRS optimization problem can be denoted the following way:

(2-8)   subject to
$$\max_{\mu,\nu} \theta = \sum_{r=1}^{s} \mu_r y_{ro} - \mu_0$$

$$\sum_{i=1}^{m} v_i x_{io} = 1$$
$$\sum_{r=1}^{s} \mu_r y_{rj} \leq \sum_{i=1}^{m} v_i x_{ij} + \mu_0 e$$
$$v_i \geq 0$$
$$\mu_r \geq 0$$
$$\mu_0 \text{ unbinded}$$

The model (2-8) describes the multiplier form of the BCC model. It differs from the original CCR model through the introduction of the additional free variable μ_0. μ_0 can either be smaller than, equal to or bigger than zero. μ_0 indicates the scale level of a DMU under evaluation. Negative values of μ_0 indicate that a DMU is operating under increasing returns of scale. A value of zero indicates constant returns of scale and any positive values for μ_0 indicate decreasing returns to scale. An efficiency value of $\theta = 1$ indicates efficient DMU's. Furthermore, it is worth mentioning that a value of 0 for μ_0 always goes hand in hand with an efficiency value of 1 for the DMU under evaluation.

Bearing in mind Figure 2.4.2-1, this fact can be clarified. Only DMU B operates under CRS. All other DMU's encompass VRS. Thus a DMU can only display CRS if it is on the CRS efficiency frontier. In general, using multi dimensional models, only a limited number of DMU's reveal CRS and hence a production size at the most productive scales size (MPSS).

Analogous to the CCR model the BCC model, has a dual input orientated optimization model which slightly differs from the formulation of its CCR counterpart and which describes the envelop form:

$$\min \theta - \varepsilon \left(\sum_{i=1}^{m} s_i^- + \sum_{r=1}^{s} s_r^+ \right)$$

(2-9) subject to

$$\sum_{j=1}^{n} \lambda_j x_{ij} + s_i^- = \theta^* x_{io}$$

$$\sum_{j=1}^{n} \lambda_j y_{rj} - s_r^+ = y_{ro}$$

$$\sum_{j=1}^{n} \lambda_j = 1$$

$$\lambda_j \geq 0$$

A new feature is the convexity constraint expressed through $\sum_{j=1}^{n} \lambda_j = 1$. This constraint indicates that the sum of the weights for the benchmark partners cannot exceed unity which is crucial for the VRS assumption.

2.4.3 The slack based measurement model

In this section the slack based measure (SBM) of efficiency in data envelopment analysis developed by Tone (2001) will be briefly introduced. In contrast to the CCR and BCC models the SBM model efficiency score deals directly with the input excesses and output shortfalls of the evaluated DMU. The SBM measure is unit invariant and monotone decreasing with respect to input excess and output shortfall.

Similar to the BCC and CCR model n DMU´s with the input and output matrices $X=(x_{ij})\in \mathbb{R}^{m\times n}$ and $Y=(y_{ij}) \in \mathbb{R}^{s\times n}$ are evaluated. It is assumed that the data set is positive, i.e. $X>0$ and $Y>0$. In accordance to the CCR and BCC model, the production possibility set P is defined as $P = \{(\mathbf{x},\mathbf{y}) | \mathbf{x} \geq X\lambda,\ \mathbf{y} \leq Y\lambda,\ \lambda \geq 0\}$ where λ is a nonnegative vector in $\mathbb{R}^n$. Again, in compliance with the BCC model, for VRS $\sum_{j=1}^{n}\lambda_j = 1$. An expression for describing a certain DMU (x_0, y_0) is considered as $\mathbf{x_o} = X\lambda + \mathbf{s^-}$ and $\mathbf{y_o} = Y\lambda - \mathbf{s^+}$. The preceding two expressions point out that the input vector of DMU$_0$ is made up out of the weighted input vectors of DMU$_0$s benchmark partners plus the input excesses which is analogous for the output vector. Of course, the preceding depends on the efficiency score attained (e.g. if DMU$_0$ is efficient, it is its own benchmark partner (input orientated efficiency: $\mathbf{x_o^*} = \mathbf{x_o}\lambda_0^* + 0^-$)).

Using $\mathbf{s^-}$ and $\mathbf{s^+}$ the following index ρ is defined:

(2-10)
$$\rho = \frac{1-(1/m)\sum_{i=1}^{m} s_i^-/x_{io}}{1+(1/s)\sum_{r=1}^{s} s_r^+/y_{ro}}$$

ρ is unit invariant, monotone and $0 < \rho \leq 1$ holds. To calculate the efficiency scores the following fractional program (here: with VRS) has to be solved:

$$\min \rho = \frac{1-(1/m)\sum_{i=1}^{m} s_i^-/x_{io}}{1+(1/s)\sum_{r=1}^{s} s_r^+/y_{ro}}$$

(2-11)   subject to

$$x_0 = X\lambda + s^-$$
$$y_0 = Y\lambda - s^+$$
$$e\lambda = 1$$
$$\lambda \geq 0, \, s^- \geq 0, \, s^+ \geq 0$$

By using the same transformation as for the BCC and CCR model the SBM model can be transformed into a linear program. This topic will not be exploited here and is left for the interested reader to read in Tone (2001).

A DMU is SBM efficient for $\rho^* = 1$ (the star indicates the optimum value). This comes alongside with $s^{-*} = s^{+*} = 0$ which can be derived straight forward from the equation. For a SBM inefficient DMU (x_0, y_0) the following expressions apply[6]:

$$x_0 = X\lambda^* + s^{-*}$$
$$y_0 = Y\lambda^* - s^{+*}$$

The inefficient DMU (x_0, y_0) can improve by deleting input excesses and augmenting output shortfalls as follows:

$$x_0^* \leftarrow x_0 - s^{-*}$$
$$y_0^* \leftarrow y_0 + s^{+*}$$

The SBM model can be interpreted as the product of input and output inefficiencies. The formula for ρ (see 2-10) can be transformed to:

(2-12)
$$\rho = \left(\frac{1}{m} \sum_{i=1}^{m} \frac{x_{i0} - s_i^-}{x_{i0}} \right) \left(\frac{1}{s} \sum_{r=1}^{s} \frac{y_{r0} + s_r^+}{y_{r0}} \right)^{-1}$$

---

[6] Cooper, Seiford and Tone (2007) define that the set of indices corresponding to positive λ_j^* s is called the reference set for (x_0, y_0) (benchmark set which defines the mentors for a inefficient sales reps). There exists the possibility of multiple optimal solutions, for which the reference set is not unique. Regarding the fact that all of the possible solutions are optimal, one can choose any one of them.

On the right hand side the first term describes the relative reduction rate of input i and thus the first term corresponds to the mean reduction rate of inputs or input inefficiency. The second term of the right hand side depicts the inverse mean expansion rate of outputs which can be interpreted as output inefficiency.

It is proven by Tone (2001) that a DMU (x_0, y_0) is CCR *strong* efficient (Pareto-Koopmans-Efficient), if and only if it is SBM-C efficient. Thus the SBM measure of efficiency is a stricter measure than the CCR efficiency measure, if the SBM model is calculated with CRS. This stems from the fact that the SBM measure ρ includes slacks and not excludes slacks like the CCR model does.

In contrast to the CCR and BCC model the SBM model can be calculated in a non orientated way. This means that the SBM model has no output or input orientation in the non orientated case but instead minimizes the distance between the efficiency frontier and an inefficient DMU so that both, inputs and outputs, are taken into account.

In addition, the SBM model can be deployed in an input or an output orientated approach, either with CRS or VRS. However, in this thesis only the non orientated SBM model is used.

Like the CCR and BCC models do, the SBM model displays benchmark partners for the inefficient DMU´s. The impact of a benchmark partner on the inefficient DMU is indicated by λ_j.

Similar to the CCR and BCC models the dual problem of the SBM model can be formed. Solving the dual program results into the shadow prices (or virtual weights) which imply the same interpretation as their counterparts in the BCC and CCR models discussed in the previous chapters. For a detailed overview of the dual SBM program the reader is referred to Tone (2001).

Decomposing the efficiency scores

In case an optimal solution with the optimal slacks has been calculated the SBM model provides the possibility to decompose the efficiency scores into its components. To achieve this goal, the following formula has to be used with the stars symbolizing optimal values:

(2-13)
$$\rho^* = \frac{1-\sum_{i=1}^{m}\alpha_i}{1+\sum_{r=1}^{s}\beta_r}$$

where $\alpha_i = \frac{1}{m}\frac{s_i^{-*}}{x_{i0}} (i=1,...,m)$

$\beta_r = \frac{1}{s}\frac{s_r^{+*}}{y_{r0}} (r=1,...,s)$

This decomposition, which only works for the SBM models, is very useful in revealing sources and magnitudes of inefficiency, considering the respective inputs and outputs of an individual unit of a DEA sample.

2.4.4 The super efficiency model

In the models discussed so far the highest attainable efficiency score is one. As a matter of fact, there are mostly plural DMU´s which achieve this score. This fact is especially important in case the absolute number of DMU´s is close to the sum of inputs and output multiplied by three (see chapter 2.4). In such a circumstance more than half of the DMUs can turn out to be efficient. This of course can be unsatisfying since too many units are efficient and therefore conclusions can only be drawn for the relative small group of inefficient DMU´s.

To overcome this shortcoming a method for ranking the efficient units was developed. There exist two approaches. One radial super efficiency model developed by Anderson and Peterson (1993) and a super efficiency model based on the slack based measurement model developed by Tone (2002). The author will stick to Tone´s model because it incorporates slacks and therefore, gives a more detailed view on efficiency and super efficiency than the radial model does.

Basically, the idea is to delete an efficient DMU from the efficiency frontier and to test how far the new efficiency frontier lies from the original efficiency frontier. The greater the distance between the original efficient DMU and the new efficiency frontier, the greater the super efficiency of the evaluated DMU is (see Figure 2.4.4-1). The distance AZ is greater than the distance CX and therefore A is more super efficient than C.

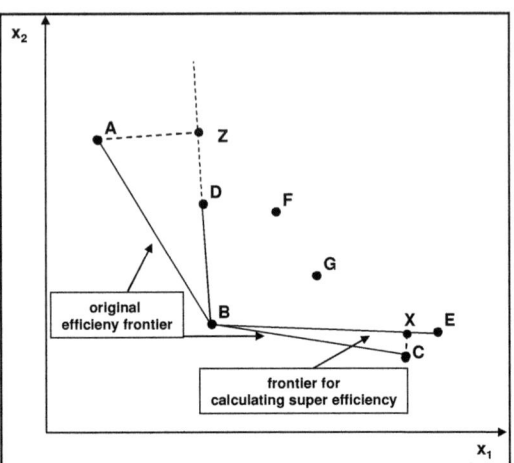

Figure 2.4.4-1: Input orientated ranking of efficient units
– basic idea

Formally Tone defines the super efficiency of a vector (x_0, y_0) as the optimal objective function value δ^* of the following program (here presented with VRS):

$$\delta^* = \min \delta = \frac{\frac{1}{m}\sum_{i=1}^{m} \frac{\bar{x}_i}{x_{i0}}}{\frac{1}{s}\sum_{r=1}^{s} \frac{\bar{y}_r}{y_{r0}}}$$

(2-14)   subject to

$$\bar{x} \geq \sum_{j=1, \neq 0}^{n} \lambda_j x_j$$

$$\bar{y} \leq \sum_{j=1, \neq 0}^{n} \lambda_j y_j$$

$$\sum_{j=1, \neq 0}^{n} \lambda_j = 1$$

$$\bar{x} \geq x_0, \quad \bar{y} \leq y_0$$

$$\bar{y} \geq 0, \quad \lambda \geq 0$$

In the case of Figure 2.4.4-1 the denominator of (2-9) is one because the output is standardized to one for all DMUs. $\bar{x}$ is the vector of the new input combination lying on the new production possibility frontier which is used to calculate the distance for the super efficiency and which excludes the (x_0,y_0) corresponding to point A. In Figure 2.4.4-1 $\overline{x}$ corresponds to point Z for DMU A. As the output y is normalized to one in Figure 2.4.4-1 it takes the value 1 for the entire program (2-9). For a numerical illustration the author refers to appendix A. The example is slightly changed from the example presented in Tone (2002).

2.4.5 The Malmquist Productivity Index

Relative efficiency is measured within one period for a sample. Therefore, the DEA method will always identify efficient and inefficient sales reps no matter what the overall development of the sample is. If overall productivity of the sample decreases (e.g. the sales reps do not sell as much anymore), DEA will still identify the efficient and the inefficient. Therefore, it is important to evaluate the productivity of the whole sample and of individual sales reps over time independently from the standard DEA approach, to track overall increases or decreases in productivity. These changes in productivity can be assessed using the so called Malmquist Productivity Index (MPI), which controls for the productivity development of the sales force based on the DEA method.

The bilateral Malmquist Productivity Index (MPI) was originally developed by Prof. Sten Malmquist. The first version of the MPI was developed to assess the production technologies of two different economies. In the context of the present thesis the MPI will be introduced as a tool to evaluate the productivity change of a DMU or sales rep between two time periods, according to Cooper, Seiford and Tone (2007). The MPI is defined as product of catch-up (CU) and frontier shift (FS) terms.

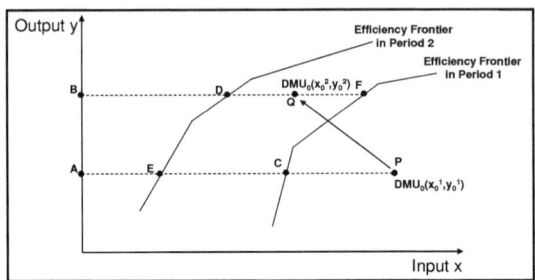

Figure 2.4.5-1: Catch up process and frontier shift from period 1 to 2 *(Source: Cooper, Seiford, Tone 2007)*

In Figure 2.4.5-1 two periods are depicted. In period 1 DMU_0 (point C) produces the output level A. In period 2 DMU_0 produces the output level B. The output level B in period 2 is higher than the output level A and DMU_0 produced level A with fewer inputs than level B in period 1. The inefficient DMU_0 moves from point P with x_0^1 and y_0^1 to point Q with x_0^2 and y_0^2 during two periods. The productivity of DMU_0 increased because it produced more output with fewer inputs. But what about the relative efficiency score though? The relative efficiency score of DMU_0 is influenced by two effects: namely the productivity increase represented by the more productive efficiency frontier in period 2 and the increasing relative efficiency in the use of inputs of DMU_0 from period one to two. If for example, the relative efficiency stays unchanged for DMU_0 from period 1 to period 2 and the efficiency frontier shifts outwards (i.e. producing output with less inputs) the DMU_0 still has the same relative distance to the outwards shifted efficiency frontier. Hence, DMU_0 produces output with less input but reaches the same efficiency score as in period 1. This would result in an MPI greater than on, indicating increased productivity. Thus, there are two *overlapping* effects which influence the productivity of DMU_0 compared with the sample: the CU and the FS.

Hence, the MPI and its decomposition give answer to the question which effects dominated and how productivity of DMU_0 developed in relation to the rest of the sample. The MPI ranges around one and the productivity of a DMU increases from one period to another if the MPI>1, decreases for MPI<1 and stays the same for MPI=1.

In terms of Figure 2.4.5-1 the CU process can be written as

$$CU = \frac{BD/BQ}{AC/AP} = \frac{\text{Efficiency of DMU}_0\ (x_0,y_0)^2 \text{ with respect to period 2 frontier}}{\text{Efficiency of DMU}_0\ (x_0,y_0)^1 \text{ with respect to period 1 frontier}} \quad (2\text{-}15)$$

Regarding efficiency a DMU is catching up to the efficiency frontier if CU>1, falling behind for CU<1 and remains unchanged for CU=1.

The frontier shift is constructed of two components. The first part implies the movement of the reference point C of the inefficient DMU_0 (x_0^1, y_0^1) to point E on the frontier of period two at the output level A. Therefore, the frontier shift at the output level A is calculated as $\phi_1 = \frac{AC}{AE}$. If the fraction ϕ_1 is expanded by AP/AP the result is

$$\phi_1 = \frac{AC/AP}{AE/AP} = \frac{\text{Efficiency of DMU}_0\ (x_0,y_0)^1 \text{ with respect to period 1 frontier}}{\text{Efficiency of DMU}_0\ (x_0,y_0)^1 \text{ with respect to period 2 frontier}} \quad (2\text{-}16)$$

The second component consists of the frontier shift at the output level B with DMU_0 (x_0^2, y_0^2) can be formulated as

$$\phi_2 = \frac{BF/BQ}{BD/BQ} = \frac{\text{Efficiency of DMU}_0\ (x_0,y_0)^2 \text{ with respect to period 1 frontier}}{\text{Efficiency of DMU}_0\ (x_0,y_0)^2 \text{ with respect to period 2 frontier}} \quad (2\text{-}17)$$

Finally the FS is defined as the geometric mean using ϕ_1 and ϕ_2 as

$$FS = \phi = \sqrt{\phi_1 \phi_2} \quad (2\text{-}18)$$

A FS>1 expresses an outwards shift of the efficiency frontier in the projection (reference) region of DMU_0 from period 1 to 2. If FS=1 or FS<1 respectively the efficiency frontier is remaining in the status quo or is regressing for the latter.

The MPI is defined as the product of CU and FS. Hence the MPI is calculated by combining (2-15), (2-16) and (2-17)

$$MPI = \frac{AP}{BQ}\sqrt{\frac{BF}{AC}\frac{BD}{AE}}_{7,} \qquad (2\text{-}19)$$

where the first term depicts the relative change in performance and the second represents the relative change in the frontier used to evaluate these performances.

With this information as background the numerical way of expressing the MPI will be evaluated in the following paragraphs. Therefore following notation for the efficiency score of DMU_0 $(x_0, y_0)^{t_1}$ in period 1 (t_1) measured by the efficiency frontier in period 2 (t_2) is presented: $\delta^{t_2}\left((x_0,y_0)^{t_1}\right)$ with $(t_2=1, 2$ and $t_1=1, 2)$.

Thus the CU process can be denoted as

$$CU = \frac{\delta^{t_2}\left((x_0,y_0)^{t_2}\right)}{\delta^{t_1}\left((x_0,y_0)^{t_1}\right)} \qquad (2\text{-}20)$$

and the frontier shift as

$$FS = \left[\frac{\delta^{t_1}\left((x_0,y_0)^{t_1}\right)}{\delta^{t_2}\left((x_0,y_0)^{t_1}\right)} \times \frac{\delta^{t_1}\left((x_0,y_0)^{t_2}\right)}{\delta^{t_2}\left((x_0,y_0)^{t_2}\right)}\right]^{\frac{1}{2}} \qquad (2\text{-}21)$$

Finally the MPI is calculated as MPI=CU*FS:

$$MPI = \frac{\delta^{t_2}\left((x_0,y_0)^{t_2}\right)}{\delta^{t_1}\left((x_0,y_0)^{t_1}\right)}\left[\frac{\delta^{t_1}\left((x_0,y_0)^{t_1}\right)}{\delta^{t_2}\left((x_0,y_0)^{t_1}\right)} \times \frac{\delta^{t_1}\left((x_0,y_0)^{t_2}\right)}{\delta^{t_2}\left((x_0,y_0)^{t_2}\right)}\right]^{\frac{1}{2}}$$

$$= \left[\frac{\delta^{t_2}\left((x_0,y_0)^{t_1}\right)}{\delta^{t_1}\left((x_0,y_0)^{t_1}\right)} \times \frac{\delta^{t_2}\left((x_0,y_0)^{t_2}\right)}{\delta^{t_1}\left((x_0,y_0)^{t_1}\right)}\right]^{\frac{1}{2}} \qquad (2\text{-}22)$$

Attributing the fact that the MPI is calculated using several efficiency scores it is necessary to calculate these individual efficiency scores with separate DEA calculations.

---

[7] for clarification: $MPI = CU*FS = \frac{BD/BQ}{AC/AP}\sqrt{\frac{AC/AP}{AE/AP}\frac{BF/BQ}{BD/BQ}} = \frac{AP}{BQ}\sqrt{\frac{AC\ AP\ BF\ BQ\ BD^2}{AP\ AE\ BQ\ BD\ AC^2}} = \frac{AP}{BQ}\sqrt{\frac{BF}{AC}\frac{BD}{AE}} = MPI$

As mentioned in previous paragraphs DEA distinguishes radial from non-radial models. Therefore, the MPI can be calculated using radial and non-radial (or slack based) measures. In this thesis the MPI will be used in the non-radial, non-orientated framework with VRS and therefore, is based on the NO-SBM-V model. Regarding the fact that there exists a possibility of infeasible results[8] calculating the MPI with the NO-SBM-V, the MPI based on the super efficiency version of the NO-SBM-V is introduced, due to the fact that the NO-SuperSBM-V always results in a feasible solution and therefore has a finite minimum in any returns to scale environment (see Tone (2002)).

Numerical the calculation of the MPI is denoted as (NO-SBM-V) for s=1, 2 and t=1, 2:

(2-23)
$$\delta^s\left((x_0, y_0)^t\right) = \min_{\varphi, \psi, \lambda} \frac{1 - \frac{1}{m}\sum_{i=1}^{m}\varphi_i}{1 + \frac{1}{q}\sum_{r=1}^{q}\psi_r}$$

$$(1-\varphi_i)x_{i0}^t = \sum_{j=1}^{n}\lambda_j x_{ij}^s \quad (i = 1,\ldots,m)$$

$$(1+\psi_r)y_{r0}^t = \sum_{j=1}^{n}\lambda_j y_{rj}^s \quad (r = 1,\ldots,q)$$

$$e\lambda = 1$$

$$\lambda \geq 0, \varphi \geq 0, \psi \geq 0$$

with $\varphi_i = s_i^-/x_{i0}^t$ and $\psi_r = s_r^+/y_{r0}^t$. In case the solutions of (2-23) are found infeasible, the NO-SuperSBM-V model is applied which can be denoted as

(2-24)
$$\delta^s\left((x_0, y_0)^t\right) = \min_{\varphi, \psi, \lambda} \frac{1 + \frac{1}{m}\sum_{i=1}^{m}\varphi_i}{1 - \frac{1}{q}\sum_{r=1}^{q}\psi_r}$$

$$(1+\varphi_i)x_{i0}^t = \sum_{j=1}^{n}\lambda_j x_{ij}^s \quad (i = 1,\ldots,m)$$

$$(1-\psi_r)y_{r0}^t = \sum_{j=1}^{n}\lambda_j y_{rj}^s \quad (r = 1,\ldots,q)$$

$$e\lambda = 1$$

$$\lambda \geq 0, \varphi \geq 0, \psi \geq 0$$

---

[8] For the problem with infeasible result the reader is referred to Cooper, Seiford and Tone (2007). Due to the application of the NO-SuperSBM-V the problems occurring with the NO-SBM-V model are solved.

Hence, an MIP>1 indicates an increase in total factor[9] productivity of DMU_0 from period 1 to 2. If MIP<1 or MIP=1 the total factor productivity decreases and remains in the status quo for the latter.

In Figure 2.4.5-2 an example of an ideal optimization process highlights the possibilities of the MPI. It is assumed that the management detected an inefficient DMU in period 1, which shall be developed and improved towards efficiency over the subsequent periods.

For this single, exemplary DMU, the productivity change and efficiency score, which both are displayed on the ordinate are given for ten time periods. The upper line stands for the overall productivity change of a sales rep. In case the productivity change from one period to another is greater than one, the evaluated sales rep is increasing the productivity. The second line from the top represents the catch up process of the evaluated sales rep. The catch up process reflects the speed with which a sales rep approaches the efficiency frontier. The third line stands for the shift of the efficiency frontier in the projection region of the evaluated sales rep.

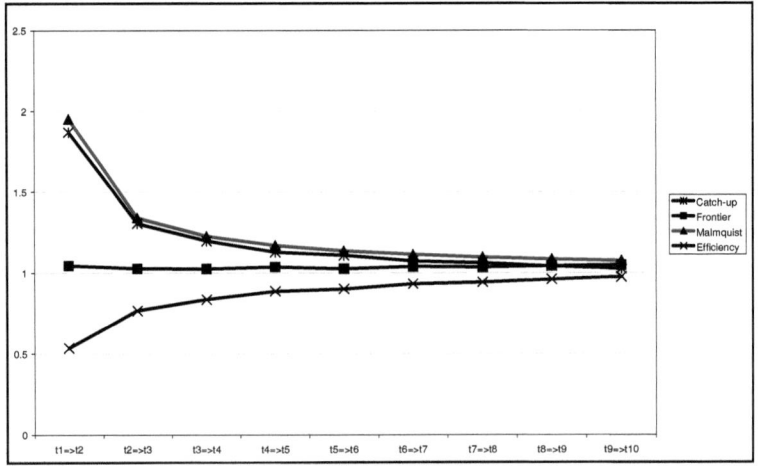

Figure 2.4.5-2: Productivity change and relative efficiency over time: example of an ideal development

---

[9] "Total factor productivity": reflects an output/input ratio which takes account of *all* outputs and *all* inputs.

In this example the frontier shift is always slightly above 1. This reflects the fact that the sales force (in the projection region) increases productivity slightly from period to period.

The lowest line depicts the development of the efficiency of a sales rep. In this example the efficiency is very low at the beginning (about 0.52). Due to a high productivity increase in the first periods (MPI of nearly 2) the relative efficiency of the sales rep increases fast. As the productivity increase slowly cools down the increase in efficiency slows down as well. This fact is also reflected by the catch up process of the evaluated sales rep, which slows down as well.

2.5 Concepts used: Management cockpit and efficiency gap

The calculations of a DEA analysis result in a great number of performance indicators and are complex. Besides the superior findings like the efficiency score, the rank of a DMU within the sample and benchmark partners of an inefficient DMU there are a lot of additional interesting aspects like, the target values, the status quo values, the percentage adjustments of each input and output dimension, the contribution of each of the dimensions to the attained efficiency score (for the SBM model), the efficiency development over time and the MPI. For the present analysis at least 40,000 different performance values were calculated which stand for a vast flood of information.

In addition to the huge amount of information the DEA is a complex mathematical method. Hence the necessity arises to present the DEA results in a simple and standardized way for understanding and implementing the crucial information.

Thus it is important to agree upon tools which summarize and communicate all important figures. A common tool are visualisations and therefore, in the next paragraph two effective visualisation concepts for communicating DEA results in a comprehensive way are presented.

2.5.1 The management cockpit

According to Meyer (1999) on a first stage the main argument for the use of a management cockpit is to support and improve the decision making quality of the management. Therefore, on a second stage, the visualisation of key performance indicators intends:

a) to increase the physically perceived, accepted and processed amount of information by the management,
b) to communicate relations between information units by meaningful aggregation and emphasising of information and
c) to support the precision and efficiency of decisions.

Considering the points listed above the management cockpit is an ideal tool to process and present the DEA results.

Due to the fact that improvements of the overall efficiency of a sample are initiated on an individual DMU level it is rational to present a management cockpit for every evaluated DMU. As far as this analysis is concerned this means that every evaluated sales rep should be assessed using the cockpit tool. Due to the great amount of DMUs in this thesis, only examples for selected sales representatives will be presented in the form of a management cockpit.

The DEA management cockpit

Figure 2.5.1-1 presents an example for a DEA management cockpit which will be discussed step by step. This example has its roots in sales management but it can be applied to every thinkable DEA application.

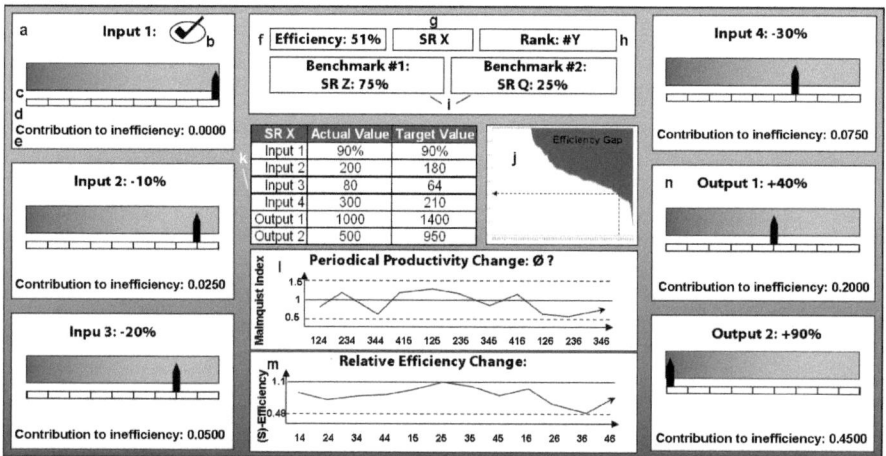

Figure 2.5.1-1: Example for a management cockpit in DEA

a) The boxes on the left and the right depict the different input and output dimensions and their characteristics. During the analysis, different input and output mixes in five separate DEA versions are evaluated and therefore, depending on the amount of inputs and outputs used, some boxes may stay blank or represent differing dimensions. Changes in the meaning of a box can be noticed due to different titles.

b) Next to the title of a box the optimal percentage change in the specific dimension is displayed. In case a sales rep is using an optimal level of a dimension in the status quo no change is needed in that category and, therefore, the box implies a checkmark next to the box title.

c) This bar is shaded from dark to light and the position of the arrow visualizes the percentage change recommended for that dimension in comparison to the other dimensions. In the lighter part of the bar only small adjustments are necessary for reaching an optimal status in that dimension, and, in the dark part strong improvements are indicated.

d) This narrower bar is separated into nine little rectangles. Each rectangle represents 10% optimization potential. A maximum of 90% optimization potential can be displayed in this way, which is sufficient for about 95% of the sales reps.

e) If the SBM model is applied the contribution to inefficiency of the specific dimension is denoted according to equation (2-13).

f) This box presents the efficiency score a sales rep achieved with in the sample. In case of the SBM model the super efficiency scores are displayed. The reason for the presentation of the super efficiency score on the one hand is to present the opportunities of ranking efficient units unmistakable

g) Here the sales rep under evaluation is depicted.

h) The rank considering the efficiency score within the sample is displayed in this box.

i) These two boxes imply the benchmark partners DEA calculated for the inefficient sales rep. In case the model is calculated with the VRS assumption, the sum of λ results in unity (see equation (2-9)) and, therefore, the values for λ correspond to percentages. These percentages correspond to the importance of an efficient unit as mentor for the unit evaluated in the cockpit. The higher the percentage, the more important an efficient sales rep is, for evaluating an inefficient sales rep. For feasibility reasons the boxes only display the two most important benchmarks. However, if the CRS assumption is assigned to the DEA model the sum of λ must not be equal to unity and therefore the λ, values do not correspond to percentages as they do for the VRS case (see equation (2-3)). Thus the importance of an efficient sales rep as benchmark partner for an inefficient unit is calculated as portion of its own λ in relation to the sum of λs of the other efficient sales reps in the benchmark set of the inefficient unit. Then the importance of the benchmarking partners can be displayed as percentages again. Things differ if the evaluated sales rep achieves an efficient status. In that case no benchmark partner for the sales rep under evaluation is needed because the efficient status is reached and, hence, the efficient sales rep is benchmark to itself. Therefore in the left one of the two boxes additional information will be added displaying the frequency of the evaluated sales rep in the benchmark sets of inefficient sales rep and, furthermore, the "impact factor" is calculated. The impact factor is calculated by summing up all the λ belonging to an efficient sales rep. As explained, the λ represent the importance of a sales rep as benchmark to others. Therefore the sum of λ s of an efficient sales rep shows the overall importance of a sales rep compared to the other efficient units. Hence, both the frequency and the impact factor can be ranked and the higher both of the ranks are the more important a sales rep is as mentor within the sample for inefficient sales reps.

j) This box presents the visualisation of the rank of a sales rep within the sample. This visualisation is called the "efficiency gap" and will be given further attention in the upcoming sub chapter.

k) This table displays the status quo (or actual value in the initial situation) and the optimal target values calculated by DEA for all dimensions. In case a sales rep reaches the target values in every dimension, an efficient status would be achieved in case the rest of the sample would remain unchanged.

l) This box displays the MPI for the sales rep under evaluation (see chapter 2.4.5 for details). Due to the occurrence of infeasible solution (see Cooper, Seiford and Tone 2007) when calculating the MPI on the bases of the NO-SBM-V model, the MPI is calculated on the basis of the NO-SuperSBM-V model. In case the MPI line is above one, the total factor productivity of the sales rep under evaluation is increasing and if it is below one, the productivity is decreasing. Furthermore, the average productivity increase over the whole time period is depicted. A good sales rep would be characterized by a MPI line, being mainly above one across time. The extent of the productivity change from period to period is indicated on the ordinate axis. The shift of periods is displayed on the abscissa axis. For example the number **234** on the abscissa stands for the change form quarter **2** to quarter **3** 200**4** and the number **126** stands for the change form quarter **1** to quarter **2** 200**6.** Hence, from the fourth quarter

2005 to the first quarter 2006 (416) the total factor productivity of the sales rep in this example increased slightly because the MPI line is above one.

m) The relative efficiency scores for each of the periods are calculated and presented in this box. The chart displays the development of the relative efficiency over time. The efficiency scores are calculated with the NO-SuperSBM-V model in the case of the SBM model due to rank the efficient units and due to the fact that the MPI is calculated on the basis of the NO-SuperSBM-V because of the already explained circumstances. If the CCR or BCC model is applied the "regular" efficiency scores are displayed with the upper bound of 1. On the ordinate axis the attained efficiency score is displayed and on the abscissa the different time periods are depicted. For example the number 34 addresses quarter **3** 200**4** and the number 26 the quarter **2** 200**6**

n) The output dimensions with its specific characteristics like the optimal percentage increases are presented in the output boxes.

The preceding lines provided the information on how to interpret the management cockpit. In this thesis the management cockpit is worked with in every DEA version (input and output arrangement) and model (CCR, BCC or SBM) to present a comprehensive overview on the selected sales reps. The impact of different DEA outcomes on each sales rep can then be compared using the cockpit. Last but not least and most important, the cockpit leads to recommendations on how to improve the performance of the evaluated sales rep.

2.5.2 The efficiency gap

The basic idea behind the efficiency gap is to visualize the distance between the efficient status and the inefficient status by ranking the DMUs. The larger the efficiency gap is the more the sample has to improve to reach an efficient status. The advantage of the efficiency gap is that it provides quick and precise information of the efficiency status of a sample. By comparing two efficiency gaps of the same sample for different periods
a decision maker can directly see changes regarding the whole sample and can see which DMUs climbed up and which DMUs lost ranks.

If different DEA versions and models are tested for the same period and sample, the efficiency gap gives information on how strict a specific version or model is regarding the efficiency score. In general, the discriminating power of a DEA version or model increases with decreasing average efficiency and an increasing standard deviation (SD). The average efficiency and the SD are very much dependent on the number of inputs and outputs chosen in relation to the size of the sample (see introduction of chapter 2.4).

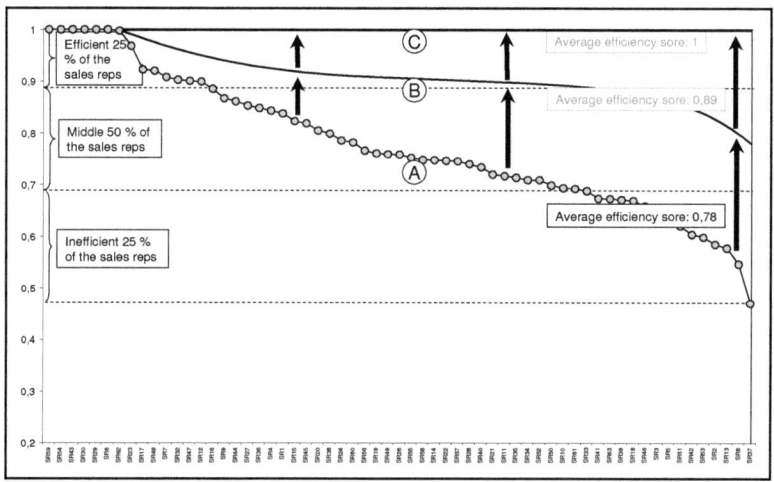

Figure 2.5.2-1: Example of an efficiency gap illustration

In Figure 2.5.2-1 the sample is divided into four quartiles. Both the first and the fourth quartile represent a single group and the second and the third quartile put together to make a third group. The allocation of a DMU to one of these groups depends solely on its efficiency score. Members of the efficient 25% group are those 15 DMUs with the highest efficiency scores out of a total of 61 DMUs. The middle 50% group accounts for those DMUs which do not reach the efficient 25% due to the fact that their efficiency score is not high enough. The 15 DMUs with the lowest efficiency score are members of the inefficient 25% group. This classification into three groups is helpful to detect underlying trends within the sample. Statements like "the inefficient 25% are very bad in the use of input x compared to the efficient 25%" are possible and can be valuable information to the management.

Therefore, the efficiency gap can be viewed as a starting point for an analysis, on a more general level, regarding underlying trends which influence the different efficiency scores of the groups.

These differences in the use of input and output dimensions between efficient and less efficient groups will be detected with the use of the so called *Mann-Whitney-U-Test* which is a non parametric test for assessing whether two samples of observations come from the same distribution. The null hypothesis is that the two samples are drawn from a single population, and, therefore, that their probability distributions are equal. The Mann-Whitney-U-Test is closely related to the t-test but with the difference that the U-Test does not require a normal distribution of the two samples compared. Because the assumption of the normal distribution does not hold for the data processed in this thesis, the U-Test is applied to detect differences between two samples (groups) regarding the input and output dimensions. Due to the fact that the U-Test is a standard tool in research, it will not be explained in detail. The interested reader is referred to Hollander and Wolfe (1999) for further details on non parametric statistical methods.

To detect these differences between the groups, the virtual weights will be analysed for the SBM model. As stated above, these weights detect the intensity with which a sales rep uses a specific input and output with respect to the objective function. In tendency efficient sales reps should be indicated by an intensive use of inputs and inefficient ones by a less intensive use. These differences will be tested for statistical significance between the efficiency groups. If, for example, the virtual weights for a dimension do not differ between groups, the sample uses this dimension in a similar intensity and therefore, this dimension than implies no strong discriminating power regarding efficiency (i.e. the leverage effect on efficiency regarding that specific dimension is more or less the same across the sample).

Unfortunately, this procedure does not work for the CCR and BCC models because a lot of the virtual weights turn out to be zero due to the existence of slack values. This fact ruins the possibility to find conclusions based on the virtual weights. As a second best solution the average group value for a dimension will be tested[10]. Ideally, this procedure should show a decreasing tendency in the average of the input dimension the more efficient a group is and

---

[10] For example the average CCD of the efficient 25% in comparison to the average CCD of the inefficient 25%.

an increasing tendency for the outputs. This approach is questionable because the efficiency is calculated as a relation between inputs and outputs. In an extreme case an efficient DMU could have ten times higher input values than the other members of the efficient 25% group but, on the other hand, ten times higher outputs. This makes the DMU efficient but would greatly increase the average input and output of the efficient 25% group and, therefore, complicates an interpretation of differences between efficiency groups based on averages of the dimensions. Due to the fact that there are no alternatives for the CCR or BCC model and due to the fact that no such extreme values exist in the data, the procedure to detect differences between the efficiency groups regarding the dimensions will be undertaken as a second best solution for the one DEA version presented in chapter 4.1.1 and 4.2.1.

Line A in Figure 2.5.2-1 represents the status quo of an exemplary sample of evaluated DMUs. The space above line A indicates the efficiency gap. The bigger the space is, the larger the improvement potential of a sample is. Caution is recommended regarding the interpretation of the efficiency gap in connection with the CCR and BCC models. The displayed efficiency scores of the sales rep do not include slack values in their calculation and hence the "real" efficiency gap should be bigger, but cannot be displayed. Things are different for the SBM model, which includes the slack values into the calculation of the efficiency scores. Thus, if the SBM model is applied for assessing the performance of DMUs the "real" (i.e. including slacks) efficiency gap is displayed.

For every manager it will be crucial to narrow the efficiency gap. A possible improvement is represented by line B where the efficiency gap would have been closed by approx. 50%. This means that the average efficiency score of the sample increased and the SD decreased. If every sales rep worked efficiently line C would be reached. This case is unrealistic but it gives an idea of the overall potential for improvements within the sample.

2.6 Software used

The calculation of the efficiency measures in this thesis is accomplished by using the "DEA-Solver-Professional-Version 5.0" (Cooper, Seiford, Tone, 2006) and "DEA-Excel-Solver" (Zhu, 2002). For data preparation and analysis in the preface of the DEA analysis "Eviews 4.1

Student Version" (2004)was applied. To detect differences between the three efficiency groups (see chapter 2.5.2) with the help of the Mann-Whitney-U-Test freely available online software for inferential statistics (VasarStats) (2007) of the Vasar College in New York was used.

3 Data, definitions and characteristics of the pharmaceutical sales process

In workshops and interviews, as part of the data mining process, several characteristics of pharmaceutical sales where elaborated. The selling process often differs from product to product and therefore the overall sales force is divided by products into several sales divisions. Each of the divisions concentrates on one product or on complementary products like insulin and drugs for erectile dysfunction.

A successful distribution strategy in one country does not mean that the same strategy works in other countries as well. Reasons for that are the size of the market, cultural differences and most important, different legislation between countries. Different market size, culture and legislation then lead to different distribution channels which in turn demand a different sales strategy. In this thesis the focus is on the insulin sales force of a big country with about 70 million residents. The author of this thesis promised confidentiality and therefore no names, whether countries or sales reps, will be provided. In addition, the current insulin sales force evaluation method used will be only presented schematically which is enough for a comparison with the DEA method.

The market situation of the sales force

The insulin market which the sales force is active in has experienced dramatic increases. Figure 3-1 displays this development. On the ordinate the amount of insulin sold is displayed in **m**ulti **mi**llion **u**nits (**MMU**) of **a**ctive **p**harmaceutical **i**ngredient (**API**). The bars reveal a steady growth with an especially big increase from 2004 to 2005. Therefore the amount of API sold should have increased for the evaluated sales force.

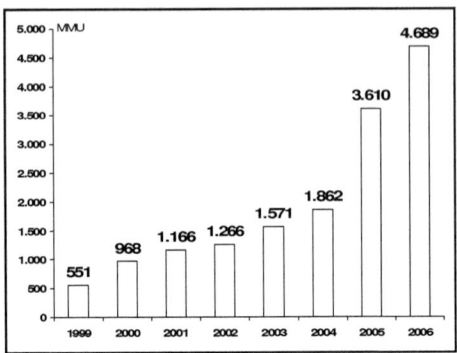

Figure 3-1: Insulin market growth from 1999 to 2006

The API of the sales force of interest increased demonstrably but as Figure 3-2 proves the share of market decreased dramatically from the first quarter 2004 to the fourth quarter 2006. Nevertheless, the absolute amount of insulin sales increased. Unfortunately the SOM decrease exactly goes in line with that time period where the strongest market growth takes place. Therefore it is crucial to identify the reasons for this decrease in market share.

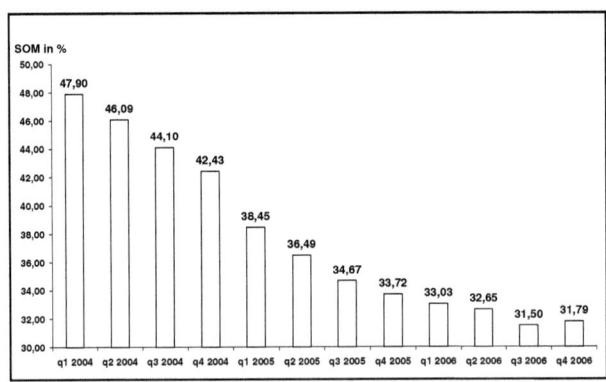

Figure 3-2: Deterioration of the share of market (SOM) from the q1 2004 to q4 2006

This decrease in market share can have several reasons. These reasons can be due to external and internal influences. Examples are:

- ➤ competitors introduce a new and better version of insulin,
- ➤ the sales force of the competitors is more efficient in targeting and closing up on customers
- ➤ the competitors sell their insulin cheaper
- ➤ the own sales force has improvement potential
- ➤ resources crucial for the sales process of insulin are redirected

With the help of the DEA method especially the improvement potential of the sales force can be uncovered due to a "best in class" comparison. The underlying question is what would happen, if every sales rep worked as good as the best in the sample. Besides others this question will be answered as part of this thesis.

3.1 Data and Definitions

The data provided by the sales management of the analyzed company were divided into measures highlighting the input side and measures highlighting the output side. The data the author was handed over originated from different sources and were arranged in different data formats. Thus, it was not arranged in a format usable for a DEA from the beginning. Henceforth, the author spent a lot of time in rearranging the data and making it usable for DEA. Finally 61 of 63 sales reps emerged as suitable for the evaluation. Two outliers (sales rep 25 and 31) had to be deleted from the sample.

The data of the input side is based on the so called "sales productivity process matrix" (SPP-matrix). In these matrices the working behavior of a sales rep is traced with the help of several different indicators which are described in chapter 3.1.1.

The data of the input side is provided by the company itself, whereas the data of the output side partly are based on company internal sales figures and are partly bought from an external company which provides data out of reach of the sales management.

The output data implies data like market shares, market size and sales volume which will be described more closely in 3.1.2.

The data ranged from January 2004 to December 2006 and will be used quarterly.

3.1.1 Sales Process Productivity (SPP) Definitions

Several different input measures were available at the beginning of the data mining process. With the experience and advice of the sales management four inputs were recommended for the use in the present analysis as a starting point to demonstrate the prospects of DEA.

Input 1: Frequency Realization (F):

Each sales representative has to visit a specific amount of customers (doctors). Each of these doctors has to be visited with an *a priori* determined frequency. Therefore the input F is defined as the percentage of **targeted customers** called on with a greater than or equal to desired frequency. This input is measured as average frequency realization per month of a quarter. The formula for this input is a percentage:

= (Number of **target customers** visited > or = to desired frequency in period) X 100
       (Total number of **targeted customers** listed in period)

The intention behind this input is that a sales rep will sell more the higher the frequency realization is. From an efficiency point of view a sales rep with a low frequency and a high sales volume would be very good because he would be able to sell a lot despite a low frequency to targeted customers. This would indicate a high quality of each visit to customers.

Input 2 and 3: Call Capacity to Customers (Doctors (CCD - input2) and Pharmacies (CCP - input3)

Before input 2 and 3 are explained in detail the term "call" and "field day (working day)" are defined. A call is a face-to-face interaction with a customer that occurs within a field day where the appropriate selling messages for relevant products are communicated.
The preferable option is to limit interactions to one customer at a time. In certain cases (i.e. hospital calls, group sells, programmes, etc.) more customers may be present. The interaction should be planned individually per customer, with clear objectives. Therefore a

"call per day" is the number of calls made by a sales representative on targeted customers per field day. Field days (working days) are the number of days a sales rep works per month. The working days do not include trainings, meetings, conferences, vacation, sick days and weekends. Working days are limited to days selling insulin and interacting directly with customers.

The *call capacity to customers (CCD, CCP)* relevant for this thesis is calculated by multiplying the average monthly "call capacity to customers per day" per quarter times the average monthly field days (working days) per quarter.

Input 2: CCD	January	February	March	Ø Quarter1 / month
Average CCD/day	9	11	10	10
Working days	17	20	20	19
CCD/month/quarter=			Input 2: CCD=	190

Table 3.1.1-1: Example for calculating the average monthly call capacity of a quarter *(analogously for CCP)*

Table 3.1.1-1 presents an example for calculating the input figures for CCD and CCP. The bold "**190**" denotes the average call capacity to customers for each month of a quarter. Therefore, in the example above, the sales rep had 190 contacts with doctors per month in the first quarter of the year. This figure normally differs from quarter to quarter. Due to the way the original data were designed, this evaluation method was chosen.

The intention behind the input "call capacity to customers" is that the sales amount of MMU insulin should increase with the amount of customers visited. But, as for the other inputs, the sales will not increase in proportion to the visits, as the sales management of the pharmaceutical company mentioned. More specific the visits underlie variable marginal returns. Like for the other inputs DEA will search for the sales rep with the best relation between calls and sales.

*Input 4: **F**ixed doctor relationships related to **T**otal doctor relationships (**F/T**):*

The input "Fixed/Total doctor relationships" expresses the percentage of sales representatives' unchanged doctor relationships within a quarter. This input is reported as average F/T rate per month in a quarter. Each sales rep visits offices of doctors. It is advantageous if the doctor in this office is always the same because then the sales rep is able to build up a personal relationship which is believed to increase the sales volume. Hence, sales reps are advised to build up long term relationships with doctors. According to common thinking, that sales rep is the best from an efficiency point of view, who sells a lot of insulin despite a low percentage of long term doctor relations. Such characteristics indicate the ability of a sales rep to quickly convince doctors without knowing them for a long time. This of course is true salesmanship.

3.1.2 Output Definitions

The output data display the results of the sales process which can be quantified into the absolute **q**uantity (**Q**) of API sold measured in MMU insulin per period, the **s**hare **o**f **m**arket (**SOM**) and the market size. This information, especially the market share, can not be calculated by the company because they do not have these figures available and therefore these data are supplied by an external consulting firm. In addition, an output called "**t**arget **r**ealization" (**TR**) is utilized for the DEA analysis. The output TR has several components and is set up by the general sales management and will be explained in detail further below.

SR X working for company A	YEAR 05	q1 2006	q2 2006
Insulin Sales in region of SR X	55,202559	17,0775163	17,4650169
by company A (sales of SR X)	14,8180115	4,28400352	4,47150387
by company B	36,015036	11,041511	10,7210107
by company C	4,36950437	1,75200175	2,27250227

Table 3.1.2-1: Excerpt of output data for a sales rep

Table 3.1.2-1 provides an excerpt of the output data for a single SR X. It displays the overall amount of MMU insulin sold by SR X and by the competitors (second line: insulin sales in region of sales rep X) for the year 2005, quarter 1 2006 and quarter 2 2006 in their specific region. The third line displays the sales of sales rep X who is working for company A in this specific region. The other two lines represent the sales of the two competitors[11]. Therefore from this table information regarding the market size a sales rep is active in and the absolute amount of insulin sold in MMU are derived. The share of market for SR X is calculated by dividing the insulin sales of SR X by the market size.

---

[11] In the insulin market of the country of interest only three competitors are active.

The output TR is a composition of different weighted measures and is set by the sales management for each sales rep. If a sales rep exceeds the sales target the output target realization takes a value greater than one. If the target is missed or hit, a value smaller than unity or unity for the latter is assigned to the sales rep as target realization. The output TR incorporates historic sales data of each sales rep in combination with the overall growth target set by the general management. Some sales reps may already sell on a level over the advised target of the general management and some on a level below that target. The individual sales targets are adjusted in the sense that poor performing sales reps (i.e. selling beneath the company average in the country) do not "drop the ball" due to unrealistically high sales targets and sales reps over performing (i.e. sales of last period already exceed the target of the next period) are released from pressure by targets that go in line with the targets of the general management.

Apparently the output TR is the most important measure within the current evaluation process for a sales rep and therefore is very useful as output measure. As one result of the analysis, that sales rep will be found who achieved the highest target realization in relation to the inputs used.

Attributing special needs for two of the DEA versions applied, an additional output had to be introduced to adjust for different market deployments. This output is introduced in the next sub chapter.

3.1.3 Reinterpreting the share of market (SOM)

For inefficient sales reps, DEA assigns optimal projections (values) for all input and output dimensions. In case the outputs "quantity MMU insulin" (Q) sold and SOM are part of the output side of a DEA analysis simultaneously, difficulties arise with the optimal target values DEA calculates.

A simple example shall clarify this fact. In case the projected optimal MMU target value for inefficient sales reps does not go in line with the projected SOM, interpretational problems come up. DEA will present projections where the target value of MMU insulin sold results in a bigger/smaller SOM than the optimal SOM projection DEA calculated. This is due to the fact that DEA maximizes the quantity sold and the market share independently of each other.

To avoid this problem the output SOM has to be redefined. At first, the question arises why to use the SOM as output in the first place then? It is true that, if all sales rep worked in identical markets, the absolute amount of MMU insulin sold would be sufficient as benchmark. Unfortunately, the markets differ very much with respect to sales potential between the individual sales reps. Hence, only focusing on the sold quantity as output, would overreach sales representatives working in a market with lower sales potential. These individuals could never reach the efficiency frontier due to their limited market size, despite being very efficient.

To avoid unfair benchmarking the market share has to be introduced as output to act as an adjusting component. DEA detects those sales reps with low insulin sales, but with high market shares and will assign them a better efficiency value as they would have achieved if DEA would have only focused on absolute insulin sales as output. Hence, introducing the market share into the calculation adjusts for misinterpretations resulting from different market deployments.

The market share can be viewed as a competition index. It shows how successful or unsuccessful a sales rep was in challenging his competitors. Taking into account that the output SOM adjusts for different market deployments, that it highlights the ability of a SR facing competition within the market and that the SOM projections are not in line with the absolute insulin sales projections, the output SOM is renamed and is included as adjusting output in upcoming DEA version with the absolute insulin sales as output and therefore is renamed to "Competition Index" (**CI**) to avoid confusions.

3.1.4 Combining inputs and outputs into one data sheet

After extracting and calculating the necessary measures the data were arranged in the following manner Table 3.1.4-1 displays for ten exemplary individuals:

DMU	(I)F	(I)CCD	(I)CCP	(I)F/T	(O)Q	(O)SOM <CI>	(O) TR
SR1	62%	200	120	83%	6,78550554	34,99%	0,961
SR2	84%	273	84	100%	6,20000551	27,91%	0,876
SR3	93%	200	140	68%	5,77850538	27,47%	0,755
SR4	75%	240	40	72%	9,48700896	35,94%	1,054
SR5	77%	200	80	85%	4,25000416	22,32%	0,757
SR6	51%	228	76	70%	6,4820059	38,93%	1,081
SR7	65%	240	100	60%	6,7145064	33,89%	1,017
SR8	90%	240	160	83%	5,12200461	28,68%	0,753
SR9	68%	240	140	71%	8,26200777	37,06%	1,045
SR10	92%	270	90	92%	8,09350741	32,71%	1,038

Table 3.1.4-1: Excerpt of the data sheet for the DEA analysis

The first column depicts the different sales reps. All columns indicated with an (I) refer to one of the four input dimensions and the columns indicated with (O) refer to output dimensions. Starting with the first column, the abbreviations refer do **D**ecision **M**aking **U**nit (**DMU**), **F**requency Realization (**F**), **C**all **C**apacity to **D**octors (**CCD**), **C**all **C**apacity to **P**harmacies (**CCP**), **F**ixed doctor relations to **t**otal doctor relations (**F/T**), **Q**uantity MMU insulin sold (**Q**), **s**hare **o**f **m**arket (**SOM**), **C**ompetition **I**ndex (**CI**) and **t**arget **r**ealization (**TR**). Table 3.1.4-1 displays part of the basic data sheet underlying all calculations for the forth quarter 2006. This data arrangement was set up for all of the quarters beginning with the first quarter 2004 and ending with the fourth quarter 2006.

Version 1	Version 2	Version 3	Version 4	Version 5
F,CCD,CCP,F/T – Q,CI	F,CCD, F/T – Q,CI	F,CCD,CCP,F/T – SOM	F,CCD,CCP,F/T – TR	F,CCD, F/T – TR

Table 3.1.4-2: Different DEA versions analysed within this thesis

Different DEA versions will be arranged (see Table 3.1.4-2) and, as part of the research, the different impacts of these versions on the efficiency scores of the sales reps will be analyzed.

3.2 Current sales representative benchmarking system

In this subsection the current sales representative evaluation system of the relevant pharmaceutical company will be highlighted. Table 3.2-1 displays in an exemplary way the evaluation system used. The input (F, CCD, CCP and F/T) and output (TR) categories are divided into different classes. Depending on which class a sales rep reached within a dimension, different amounts of points are received. For example, if a sales rep had a call capacity to doctors (CCD) of 242, 3.5 points were achieved in that dimension. Each dimension has a specific importance within the sales process. It is obvious that the output side should receive the highest weights since the concern is about sales. The weights for the different dimensions are depicted in the last column. The output side has the biggest weight of 0.7 and the input dimensions add up to a total of 0.3. The table below exactly reflects the principle how sales representatives are currently evaluated.

Points	F	Points	CCD	Points	CCP	Points	F/T	Points	TR	Dimensions	Weights
0	70%	0	220	0	80	0	70%	0	0,894	F	0,03
1,5	79%	1,5	235	1,5	100	1,5	79%	1,5	0,964	CCD	0,15
5	80%	3,5	250	3,5	120	5	80%	3,5	1,034	CCP	0,07
5	94%	4,5	265	4,5	140	5	94%	4,5	1,094	F/T	0,05
5	95%	5	270	5	160	5	95%	5	1,095	TR	0,7

Table 3.1.4-1: Evaluation system for realizations in different dimension

Applying this method to ten exemplary sales reps from the original dataset Table 3.2-2 results. With the help of the weights the total points a sales rep achieved are calculated and depicted on the far right. With 3.705 point sales rep 10 is the best. The worst sales rep is number 5 who only achieved 0.4 using the current benchmarking approach.

At this point of the thesis some important findings regarding the current evaluation system shall be mentioned:

1. the classes are set up by external and subjective evaluations
2. the points for each of the classes are set up externally and subjectively
3. the weights for the points are set up in the same way
4. all of the sales reps are lumped together in the sense that the same weights and points are assigned to all of them
5. the focus is more on effectiveness than on efficiency (see Figure 2.2.1-1)

DMU	Points	(I)F	Points	(I)CCD	Points	(I)CCP	Points	(I)F/T	Points	(O) TR	Total weighted points
SR1	0	62%	0	200	3,5	120	5	83%	1,5	0,961	1,545
SR2	5	84%	5	273	1,5	84	5	100%	0	0,876	1,255
SR3	5	93%	0	200	3,5	140	0	68%	0	0,755	0,395
SR4	1,5	75%	3,5	240	0	40	1,5	72%	4,5	1,054	3,795
SR5	1,5	77%	0	200	1,5	80	5	85%	0	0,757	0,4
SR6	0	51%	1,5	228	0	76	1,5	70%	4,5	1,081	3,45
SR7	0	65%	3,5	240	3,5	100	0	60%	3,5	1,017	3,22
SR8	5	90%	3,5	240	5	160	5	83%	0	0,753	1,275
SR9	0	68%	3,5	240	4,5	140	1,5	71%	3,5	1,045	3,365
SR10	5	92%	5	270	1,5	90	5	92%	3,5	1,038	3,705

Table 3.1.4-2: Evaluation table of ten exemplary sales reps

In terms of Figure **2.2.1-2** the performance evaluation approach applied by the company fits into class III literature approaches. These approaches take inputs and outputs into account but do not explicitly compare a salesperson with his or her peers (as DEA does), but can be rank-ordered for purpose of comparison.

At the end of this thesis the current evaluation system will be compared to the DEA results and advantages and shortcomings will be evaluated.

4 Empirical efficiency analyses

Chapter 2.1 gave an overview over the current situation in the field of sales performance evaluation focussing on DEA after 1995. As Boles et al. point out, DEA is a very promising method for sales performance evaluation because it incorporates objective and subjective measures as well as multiple inputs and outputs and therefore is advantageous compared to the methods structured in the classes I to IV (see Figure 2.2.1-2). In addition, it identifies sources and amounts of inefficiencies.

Up to now DEA has been applied to the evaluation of salesmen on a basic level which leaves space for a lot of research to be done.
Despite the fact that DEA seems to be a useful instrument in evaluating sales units, the case of inter temporal analysis remains an interesting field of research. Donthu and Yoo (1998) evaluate the efficiency of retail stores in three subsequent periods by calculating efficiency values for each year but they do not make use of a real inter temporal DEA variant. De Mateo (2006) analyses *dynamic* future developments in the case of department stores and uncovers the adjustment cost of a store for moving towards efficiency. Furthermore Chonko (2000) points out that the timing of measurement is crucial for attaining suitable DEA data.
Regarding the limited number of studies applying DEA to sales, in the empirical part of the present work, following research is proposed: in using the historic (2004-2006) data of sales personnel an inter-temporal examination of relative efficiency movements of each sales unit during subsequent periods will be undertaken.
In addition the productivity change from quarter to quarter of each sales unit will be analysed using the MPI.

Due to the progress in research and programming several different variants of DEA are available for the task of salesmen evaluation.
DEA variants like the slack based measurement model and super efficiency model are applied in addition to the standard CCR and BCC models for the case of sales evaluation.
The procedure will be as follows. In the first part of the empirical analyses the focus will be on the fourth quarter of 2006. The CCR and BCC model will be calculated and analysed for that quarter and advantages, shortcomings and differences will become clear. The SBM model will

be applied to the fourth quarter 2006 as well but in addition inter-temporal aspects will be elaborated using the MPI.

All of the analysis of the fourth quarter 2006 will be divided into a more global part where general statements regarding the whole sales force will be written and in an individual part. In the more general part the sales force is divided into three different groups (see chapter 2.5.2) which are characterized by similar efficiency scores. With the help of this division into groups, different relations between the dimensions and the efficiency scores will be highlighted for each of the groups. The individual part evaluates three exemplary sales reps to point out the different impacts of changes in the model and version on the individual sales rep performance. The three sales reps are chosen from the efficient group, the middle group and from the inefficient group.

After the results for the CCR and BCC models have been presented, the SBM model will be evaluated under an inter-temporal aspect as well.

The analysis of the fourth quarter 2006 will be similar to the CCR and BCC model but will additionally incorporate a decomposition of the inefficiency on the individual level. Furthermore, the inter-temporal analysis will reveal which effects dominate the productivity change on an individual level, the frontier shift or the catch up process. To be able to rank efficient units and due to the discussion in chapter 2.4.5 the topic of super efficiency will be elaborated as well.

The analysis begins with the presentation of the CCR model. In contrast to the five versions of the DEA SBM model the CCR and BCC models are only presented in a single version in order not to overstretch this analysis. The main differences between the three DEA variants can be evaluated using this limited setting. However, the corresponding summary at the end of the CCR and BCC chapters accounts for all five BCC and CCR versions. Chapter 4.1 evaluates the CCR model and chapter 4.2 the BCC model. Finally the inter-temporal approach based on the SBM model in chapter 4.3 is introduced.

4.1 Results of the CCR model

In this subsection the first of the three DEA models, the CCR model, is applied to evaluate the sales force. The CCR model is the basic model in DEA and all other models build up on this model in some way or another. As explained in chapter 2.4.1, the CCR model assumes constant returns to scale. In addition, the efficiency measure of the CCR model does not account for slacks. Slacks are calculated separately according to the presented two stage optimization. In this subchapter only one version will be dealt with in detail and finally the different input output arrangements calculated for the CCR model (see appendix B) will compared in a summary. The analysis reveals the impact of changes in the input and output structure on the efficiency score and for identifying an optimal DEA arrangement. The CCR model will be applied with an output orientation accounting for the fact that sales generally should be increased to increase the successes of a company. Hence the question evaluated is to which extent sales can be increased for given inputs.

4.1.1 CCR DEA Version 1 (F, CCD, CCP, F/T - Q, CI)

The first DEA version presented includes the frequency realization (F), the fixed doctor to total doctor relations (F/T), the call capacity to doctors (CCD) and to pharmacies (CCP) as inputs and the quantity of insulin sold (Q) and the competition index (CI) as outputs.

The Efficiency Gap

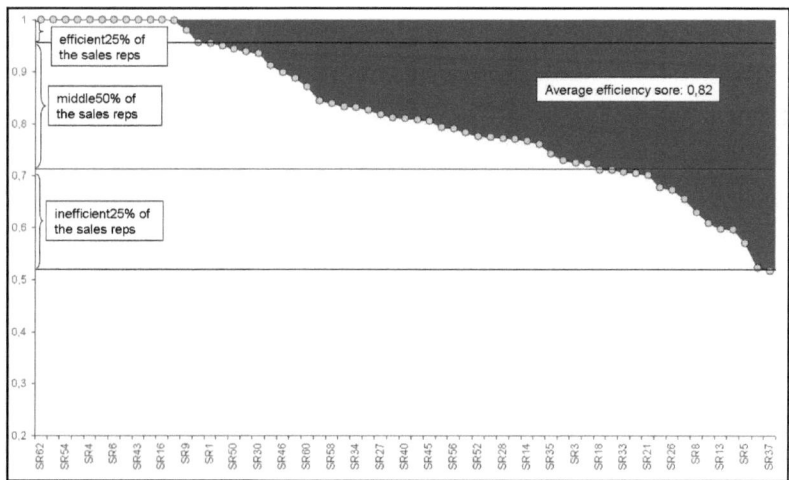

Figure 4.1.1-1: Illustration of the Efficiency Gap and of the three efficiency groups

At first the so called efficiency gap is presented by turning the attention of the reader to Figure 4.1.1-1. On the ordinate the efficiency values for each of the 61 sales reps are displayed. The higher the efficiency score is, the more efficient a sales rep is. The reader may be reminded that Figure 4.1.1-1 only depicts the radial efficiency scores and therefore slacks are not accounted for in the figure. The efficiency scores of the sample range between 0.51 and 1. The average efficiency score of the sample in this setting is 0.84. The top 25% all reach an efficient status except of two sales reps and the inefficient 25% reach from 0.51 to about 0.72.

Attributing the problems with the virtual weights and the slack values in the CCR and BCC model discussed in chapter 2.5.2 the group average for a dimension will be analyzed to detect differences between the efficiency groups regarding the dimensions. Table 4.1.1-1 shows the details. The first column refers to the input and output dimension. The second column displays the different comparisons between the efficiency groups. The third column depicts the average group value for the specific dimension and the next column the mean ranks as results of the M-W-U-Test. The next two columns present the z-value and the p-value. In this thesis the differences between the groups will be tested at a level of significance of $p \leq 5\%$.

Input/Output	Group	Group Average	Mean Rank	z-value	doublesided p-value
Frequency	efficient 25%	0.76	18.8	-1.63	0.1031
	middle 50%	0.83	25.8		
	efficient 25%	0.76	13.3	-1.37	0.1707
	inefficient 25%	0.84	17.7		
	middle 50%	0.83	23.6	0.06	0.9522
	inefficient 25%	0.84	23.3		
CCD	efficient 25%	205	19.4	-1.44	0.1499
	middle 50%	222	25.5		
	efficient 25%	205	12.8	-1.64	0.101
	inefficient 25%	238	18.2		
	middle 50%	222	22.6	-0.66	0.5093
	inefficient 25%	238	25.4		
CCP	efficient 25%	90	17.7	-2.02	0.0434
	middle 50%	107	26.3		
	efficient 25%	90	12.8	-1.64	0.101
	inefficient 25%	106	18.2		
	middle 50%	107	23.9	0.25	0.8026
	inefficient 25%	106	22.8		
F/T	efficient 25%	0.72	17.5	-2.11	0.0349
	middle 50%	0.82	26.4		
	efficient 25%	0.72	12.1	-2.07	0.0385
	inefficient 25%	0.84	18.9		
	middle 50%	0.82	23.1	-0.27	0.7872
	inefficient 25%	0.84	24.3		
Q	efficient 25%	6.99	28.5	1.73	0.0836
	middle 50%	6.15	21.1		
	efficient 25%	6.99	20.3	2.99	0.0028
	inefficient 25%	5.14	10.7		
	middle 50%	6.15	17.7	-2.04	0.0414
	inefficient 25%	5.14	26.3		
CI	efficient 25%	0.36	30.7	2.51	0.0121
	middle 50%	0.33	20		
	efficient 25%	0.36	22.4	4.25	<.0001
	inefficient 25%	0.27	8.6		
	middle 50%	0.33	28.3	3.5	0.0005
	inefficient 25%	0.27	13.5		

Table 4.1.1-1: Differences between the efficiency groups regarding the input and output dimensions

> The mean ranks of the input F between the efficiency groups do not differ significantly. Therefore, using this method, no difference between the efficiency group and the characteristic of the input F exists.

> There is no significant difference in the mean ranks of CCD between the groups in this setting. This means that CCD cannot be taken as explanation for differences in efficiency realization among the groups *in this setting*, because the sales reps all use a similar amount of CCD.

> The mean ranks of the input CCP differ significantly between the efficient and middle group. This finding provides the information that the efficient 25% use less CCP than the middle group does, which helps to detect one of the reasons why the efficient 25% are more efficient than the rest. The inefficient 25% nearly differ significantly and a significant difference would be probably detected with an increased sample.

> The input F/T is characterized by significant differences between the three groups. Therefore the efficient group is better than the other two groups in turning the fixed doctor relations into output. This again is a reason for differences in efficiency.

> The output Q differs significantly between the top and the low and the middle and the low group. The mean ranks of the top and the middle group differ significantly and an increased sample size would probably lead to significant differences. Hence the output Q is an important characteristic for distinguishing inefficient from efficient sales reps, where efficient ones sell more than inefficient ones.

> The way the different groups cope with their competitors differs very significantly. The more efficient a sales rep is the he can face competition.

For each DEA version and model the results of the above analysis differ as will be presented in later chapters. However, this method is a possible approach to detect how input and output levels differ with respect to the achieved efficiency score.

By calculating optimal targets for each input and output category, the opportunity costs of inefficiency for this DEA arrangement are revealed. If the status quo of quarter 4 2006 is compared with the optimal situation for the fourth quarter 2006 following table results:

CCR DEA	Current Value	Target Value	Delta %
Ø Frequency	81%	80%	-1%
CCD	13517	13379	-1%
CCP	6245	5442	-13%
Ø F/T	80%	78%	-2%
Q	372.70	471.47	27%
SOM	31.79%	37.65%	5.85%

Table 4.1.1-2: Optimal projection – opportunity cost of inefficiency

The target values displayed in Table 4.1.1-2 represent optimal values incase all sales reps work efficient. This of course cannot be achieved to 100% but it gives an idea of the potential within the sales force. Despite the output orientation of the model especially the input CCP has to be decreased. This is due to the existence of slacks which are not represented in the radial efficiency measure assigned to each sales rep. The input CCP therefore seems to be the one with the greatest adjustment needs when it comes to selling insulin. If all sales reps would work efficient the insulin sales would rise by 27% which represents a market share increase of 5.85%.

Benchmarking of individual sales reps

To demonstrate the impacts of changes in the model and versions three representative sales reps are chosen; one from the efficient group, one from the middle group and one from the inefficient 25%. From the top group sales rep 4, from the middle group sales rep 28 and from the weak group sales rep 42 are selected. The data set for all sales reps is presented in the appendix B.

The results for sales rep 4 are displayed in Figure 4.1.1-2. Within the setting of this chapter 4.1.1, sales rep 4 is 100% efficient and therefore is ranked number one. Because SR 4 is efficient no benchmark is necessary for evaluating SR 4. In fact SR 4 is mentioned 17 times in the benchmark set of inefficient sales reps. The sum of λ (see chapter 2.4) which depicts the importance or impact as benchmark partner for the sample amounts to 4.9 and hence SR 4 is ranked #8 regarding the impact factor. In addition all input categories are green (green=optimal). The output side is green as well. Therefore the relation between inputs and outputs is chosen in an optimal way by SR4. This fact is additionally visible from the table that depicts the current and projected values in the centre of the cockpit. Both, current and projected values of SR 4´s inputs and outputs are the same and therefore SR 4 is not only weak efficient (radial efficient, but with slacks) but also strong efficient in the sense of Pareto-Koopmans-Efficiency (no slacks present).

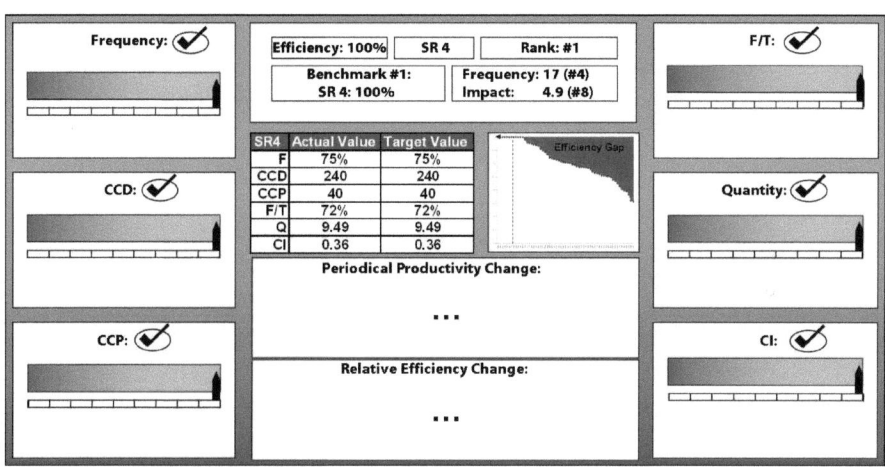

Figure 4.1.1-2: KPI-Cockpit for SR 4

Figure 4.1.1-3 depicts the results for SR 28 from the middle group. SR 28 achieved an efficiency score of 77%, has no slacks and is ranked #39. Hence the proportional output increase can be directly seen from the radial efficiency score. As explained above the CCR output orientated efficiency score ϕ ranges between one and $+\infty$ [12]. To transform the output orientated efficiency score to a score ranging between zero and one, the output orientated efficiency score is recalculated by dividing one by the output orientated score. Taking a closer look on the radial output orientated score of 129% [13] it becomes evident that SR 28 could increase the output by 29% for the given amount of inputs. Due to the fact that SR 28 has no slacks on the input or output side, the input side is green and the output side should be increased radially by 29%.

Benchmark partner for SR 28 are SR 32 with an impact of 39% and SR 48 with an impact of 31%. Therefore SR 28 should take a close look on the way of operation of these two sales reps for improvement.

---

[12] $1/\theta = \phi$, with $0 < \theta \leq 1$
[13] $1/0.77 = 1.29$

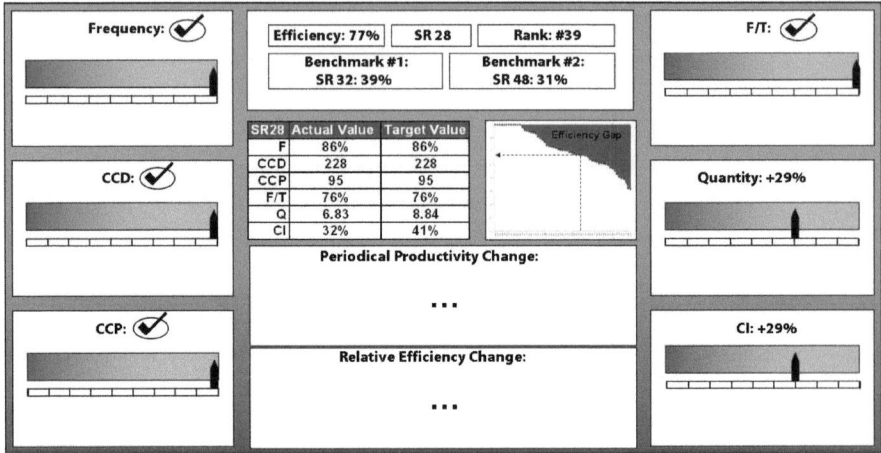

Figure 4.1.1-3: KPI-Cockpit for SR 28

The results for SR 42, who is a member of the least efficient 25%, are presented in Figure 4.1.1-4. SR 42 reached an efficiency score of 59% and is ranked on the 58th position. The benchmark partners for SR 42 are SR 44 to 65% and SR 47 to 16%. The input side is green and the output side can be expanded radial by almost 68%. The output orientated efficiency score ϕ accounts to 167.7%. In addition SR 42 has a slack in the output quantity sold. This leads to an additional recommended output increase of insulin sold by 175%. In total the optimal output increase amounts to 243%. This output dimension is the main weakness of SR 42. It is far too low. Therefore two conclusions could be drawn:

- SR 42 is a weak performer due to bad salesmanship (i.e. weak factor productivity)
- or SR 42 was assigned a territory with low potential by the general management

The weak competition index which could be improved by 67% supports the first conclusion. Therefore SR 42 should leave the company on the basis *of this DEA version.*

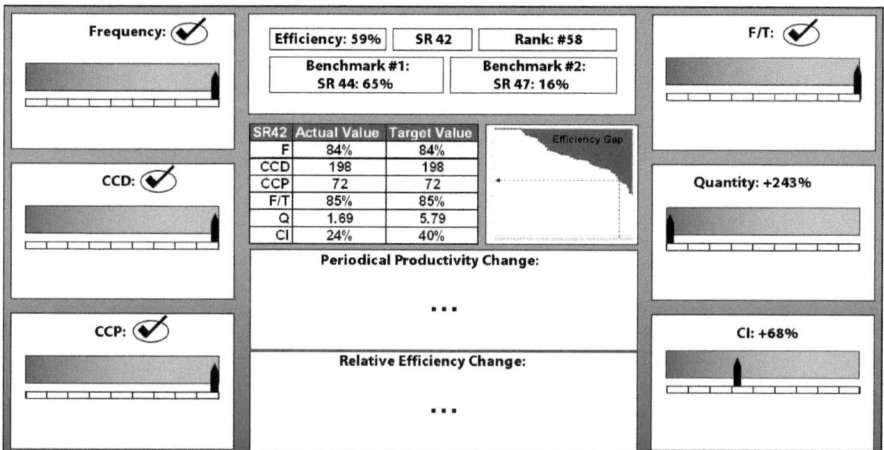

Figure 4.1.1-4: KPI-Cockpit for SR 42

4.1.2 Summary of the CCR DEA model

In chapter 4.1.1 one CCR DEA version for sales force evaluation was presented. As a matter of fact the focus in this thesis lies on the inter-temporal SBM model. Therefore only one CCR version is presented in detail which is enough to highlight the main characteristics of this model. For a complete overview all five CCR versions where calculated and the main results are summarized in this chapter. Figure 4.1.2-1 depicts the efficiency gaps for all of the different DEA settings.

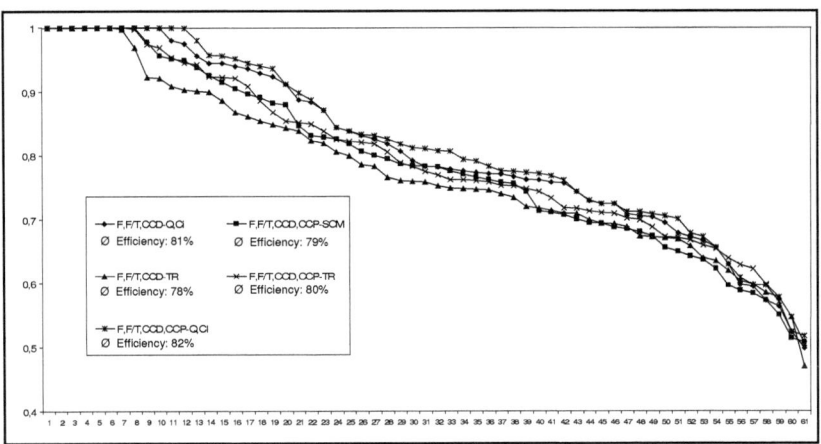

Figure 4.1.2-1: Efficiency gap comparison of the different CCR DEA versions

It is clearly visible that the four dimensional setting with the F, F/T and CCD as inputs and TR as output (line with triangles) results into the strictest efficiency measure because the triangle line is the lowest. This finding is additionally supported by the lowest average efficiency score for this setting of 78%. Figure 4.1.2-1 reveals the tendency that a rising amount of inputs and outputs for a given number of DMUs results into increasing efficiency scores. The highest average efficiency score of 82% (line with stars) is assigned to the six dimensional setting with F, F/T, CCD, CCP as inputs and Q and CI as outputs.

The summaries for the sales reps 4, 28 and 42 are presented in Tables 4.1.2-1 to 3. The percentage values in the input and output lines are the percentage decreases (for inputs) and increases (for outputs) from the status quo. The benchmark rows display the impact of the different efficient SRs as mentoring partner for the evaluated sales rep in the specific setting. The columns show the different DEA settings. The last row depicts the efficiency score of the evaluated sales rep in each of the DEA variants.

SR 4		(1) F,F/T,CCD,CCP-Q,CI	(2) F,F/T,CCD-Q,CI	(3) F,F/T,CCD,CCP-SOM	(4) F,F/T,CCD,CCP-TR	(5) F,F/T,CCD-TR
Inputs	F	0.00%	0.00%	0.00%	0.00%	0.00%
	TTD	0.00%	0.00%	0.00%	0.00%	0.00%
	TTP	0.00%	0	0.00%	0.00%	0
	DR	0.00%	~	0.00%	0.00%	~
Outputs	Q	0.00%	0.00%	~	~	~
	CI	0.00%	0.00%	~	~	~
	TR	~	~	~	0.00%	18.59%
	SOM	~	~	0.00%	~	~
Benchmarks	SR29	~	~	~	~	0.53
	SR54	~	~	~	~	0.06
	SR59	~	~	~	~	0.55
Efficiency		100%	100%	100%	100%	84%

Table 4.1.2-1: Summarized results for SR4

Sales rep 4 is inefficient only in the setting (5) with F, F/T, CCD as inputs and TR as output. Therefore only in this setting benchmark partners are assigned to SR 4 and an output expansion of 18.59% is calculated. Because of the fact that the benchmark weights have not got to add up to 1 in the CCR model, the benchmark weights are not displayed as percentages. They only give the value of the scalar with which one has to multiply the output vector of the benchmark partners to reach the efficient status of SR 4[14].

The situation for SR 28 is very different. The efficiency scores of SR 28 range between 74% (5) and 77% (1) and (2). SR 28 nearly never has got a slack on the input side except in version (2) in F/T. This indicates that SR28 is using no excessive amounts of inputs. The fact that the applied DEA model is output orientated, explains why radial reductions on the input side never occur. In version (1) and (4) the optimal output can be reached by radial expansion and henceforth it is straightforward that there are no slacks on the output side. The other versions are without slacks on the output side as well.

Turning the attention to the benchmark partners in the different versions no dominant benchmark is detectable. Table 4.1.2-2 displays that SR 30 in version (5), SR 16 and SR 32

---

[14] For this case: projection of TR for SR 4: 0,53*0,99+0,06*1,1+0,55*1,18=1,25

in version (1) and (2) and SR 54 in version (5) and (4) are the most important for the evaluation for SR 28 because they have the biggest impact on the evaluation of the inefficiency of SR 28.

SR28		(1) F,F/T,CCD,CCP-Q,CI	(2) F,F/T,CCD-Q,CI	(3) F,F/T,CCD,CCP-SOM	(4) F,F/T,CCD,CCP-TR	(5) F,F/T,CCD-TR
Inputs	F	0.00%	0.00%	0.00%	0.00%	0.00%
	TTD	0.00%	0.00%	0.00%	0.00%	0.00%
	TTP	0.00%	~	0.00%	0.00%	~
	DR	0.00%	-21.26%	0.00%	0.00%	0.00%
Outputs	Q	29.43%	9.66%	~	~	~
	CI	29.43%	9.66%	~	~	~
	TR	~	~	~	31.17%	35.13%
	SOM	~	~	32.34%	~	~
Benchmarks	SR6	0.12	~	0.28	~	~
	SR16	0.02	0.57	~	~	~
	SR32	0.45	0.30	~	~	~
	SR30	~	~	~	0.11	0.71
	SR43	0.18	~	0.15	0.24	~
	SR44	~	~	0.31	~	~
	SR47	~	~	0.17	~	~
	SR48	0.36	~	~	~	~
	SR54	~	~	~	0.28	0.29
	SR59	~	~	~	0.48	0.03
	SR62	~	0.10	0.33	~	~
Efficiency		77%	77%	75%	76%	74%

Table 4.1.2-2: Summarized results for SR28

The next table presents the summary for SR 42. The efficiency scores of SR 42 range between 57% in version (2) and 65% in version (4). An interesting fact is that the worst efficiency score occurs in version (4). SR 28 had the worst efficiency score in version (5). Therefore, when it comes to target realization, SR 42 is better off compared to SR 28 in version (5) because the distance between the two efficiency scores is smaller. Evaluating Q and CI as outputs (version 2), SR 42 falls back compared to SR 28.

In all versions no reductions on the input side are necessary and therefore no slacks exist. On the output side there are immense increases calculated to reach an efficient status. The amount of insulin sold should be expanded by over 240% in version (1) and (2). In addition the way SR 42 faces competition has to be changed significantly compared to the efficient SRs. Turning the attention to version (3) CI has to be improved by 67% on the basis of the status quo. This goes in line with the heavy increase of Q in (1) and (2). In addition SR 42 is far below the optimal target realization as indicated by the results of versions (5) and (4). The main benchmark partners for SR 42 are SR 4, SR 43 and SR 44.

SR 42		(1) F,F/T,CCD,CCP-Q,CI	(2) F,F/T,CCD-Q,CI	(3) F,F/T,CCD,CCP-SOM	(4) F,F/T,CCD,CCP-TR	(5) F,F/T,CCD-TR
Inputs	F	0.00%	0.00%	0.00%	0.00%	0.00%
	TTD	0.00%	0.00%	0.00%	0.00%	0.00%
	TTP	0.00%	0	0.00%	0.00%	0
	DR	0.00%	~	0.00%	0.00%	~
Outputs	Q	243.40%	299.15%	~	~	~
	CI	67.69%	74.48%	~	~	~
	TR	~	~	~	52.83%	65.59%
	SOM	~	~	67.69%	~	~
Benchmarks	SR4	0.05	~	0.05	0.33	~
	SR6	0.13	~	0.13	~	~
	SR30	~	~	~	~	0.18
	SR43	~	0.63	~	0.57	0.76
	SR44	0.67	~	0.67	~	~
	SR47	0.17	~	0.17	~	~
	SR48	~	0.39	~	~	~
	SR54	~	~	~	0.07	0.15
	SR59	~	~	~	0.10	~
	SR62	~	0.08	~	~	~
Efficiency		59%	57%	59%	65%	60%

Table 4.1.2-3: Summarized results for SR42

Table 4.1.2-4 displays the frequencies and Table 4.1.2-5 the impact (summed up benchmark weights λ_j of efficient sales reps from the envelop problem) of efficient sales reps in the benchmark sets of inefficient sales reps for different DEA versions. From a managerial point of view these two tables show the importance of efficient sales reps as mentors for inefficient sales reps. The higher the frequency **and**[15] the impact value of an efficient sales rep are, the more important this specific sales rep is for the improvement of the sales force. Depending on the DEA version applied the management can detect which sales rep of the efficient group is necessary for training the inefficient reps. If a sales rep is detected as important mentor for inefficient ones, the sales target of this specific efficient sales rep should be readjusted with regard to the fact, that this rep will not spent so much time in the field, due to the obligations

---

[15] A high frequency accompanied by a very low impact value does not indicate a high importance of an efficient sales rep. In contrast, a high impact value in the BCC model indicates higher influence as mentor for inefficient sales reps. The best combination, with respect to the importance for the improvement of the overall sales force, is a high frequency with coming along with a high impact value.

as mentor for inefficient sales reps. Therefore, the sales management should take these tables into account when setting up sales targets for the next period.

SR 43 is mentioned 175 times followed by SR 54 with 114 times. SR 43 and SR6 are mentioned in every DEA variant as benchmark partner which indicates that this sales rep is in the efficient group in each variant. SR 29 is only mentioned 10 times and is only efficient in version (5) and (4) with TR as output. SR 30 is in a similar situation as SR 29 because only advantages in the measure target realization. SR 32 for instance is only efficient when looking at the amount of insulin sold and the CI as output.

Sales Reps	(1) F,F/T,CCD,CCP-Q,CI	(2) F,F/T,CCD-Q,CI	(3) F,F/T,CCD,CCP-SOM	(4) F,F/T,CCD,CCP-TR	(5) F,F/T,CCD-TR	Sum
SR4	17	5	9	18	0	49
SR6	24	12	34	7	7	84
SR16	16	29	0	0	0	45
SR29	0	0	0	4	6	10
SR30	0	0	0	30	47	77
SR32	34	34	0	0	0	68
SR43	35	40	31	39	30	175
SR44	9	0	21	0	0	30
SR47	9	0	16	0	0	25
SR48	15	17	23	0	0	55
SR54	15	18	0	39	42	114
SR59	3	2	2	42	25	74
SR62	15	22	26	0	0	63
Sum	192	179	162	179	157	869

Table 4.1.2-4 Frequency of efficient benchmarks

Table 4.1.2-5 depicts the cumulated benchmark weights of an efficient sales rep for each DEA version. Again SR 43 is the most important summed up overall versions but not always the most important within a single DEA version. Interestingly SR 30 is the second important, despite the fact that SR 30 is only efficient in version (5) and (4). This is due to the fact that SR 30 has a very high impact as mentor, in the cases where SR 30 is efficient. The least important is SR 29 which goes hand in hand with the finding of Table 4.1.2-4.

Table 4.1.2-6 summarizes the insulin output projections of each DEA version. These absolute insulin sales are transformed into the optimal market share attainable based on the status quo. The projected amount of Q sold varies between 471 MMU (+26%) and 502 MMU (+34%)

depending on the DEA version applied. The corresponding market share projections vary between 37,66% (+5,87 % points) and 40,1% (+8,3% points)

Sales Reps	(1) F,F/T,CCD,CCP-Q,CI	(2) F,F/T,CCD-Q,CI	(3) F,F/T,CCD,CCP-SOM	(4) F,F/T,CCD,CCP-TR	(5) F,F/T,CCD-TR	Sum
SR4	4.90	1.96	2.85	5.90	0	15.61
SR6	7.15	4.55	13.26	3.89	2.93	31.77
SR16	6.84	27.61	0	0	0	34.44
SR29	0	0	0	2.62	3.71	6.33
SR30	0	0	0	24.41	21.17	45.59
SR32	9.63	9.55	0	0	0	19.18
SR43	11.13	14.72	11.91	13.95	9.94	61.65
SR44	3.24	0	10.10	0	0	13.34
SR47	2.70	0	4.73	0	0	7.43
SR48	5.97	0	11.90	0	0	17.87
SR54	5.66	6.38	0	14.80	17.16	44.00
SR59	1.34	1.32	1.09	14.02	9.77	27.54
SR62	5.50	7.61	10.02	0	0	23.13
Sum	64.04	73.69	65.86	79.60	64.68	347.87

Table 4.1.2-5: Impact factors of the efficient sales reps in the different CCR DEA version

Finally the CCR version of DEA indicates a potential market share increase to at least 37.66 % (for quarter 4 2006) by making the inefficient sales reps work as good as the efficient ones in the sample.

CCR DEA Version	Unit	Actual Value	Target Value	Delta
F, F/T, CCD, CCP-Q, CI	Q	372,70	471,47	26,50%
	SOM	31,79%	37,66%	5,87%
F, F/T, CCD-Q, CI	Q	373	479	28,66%
	SOM	31%	38%	6,93%
F, F/T, CCD, CCP-TR	Q	372,70	489,44	31,32%
	SOM	31,79%	39,10%	7,30%
F, F/T, CCD-TR	Q	372,70	501,92	34,67%
	SOM	31,79%	40,10%	8,30%
F, F/T, CCD, CCP-SOM	Q	372,70	480,46	28,91%
	SOM	31,79%	38,38%	6,59%

Table 4.1.2-6: Overall insulin and market share increases in case of efficient operation of all sales reps

Chapter 4.1 presents an overview over possible DEA settings, calculated by using the output orientated CCR method.

Critical annotations on the CCR model

A critical aspect is the fact that all of the CCR models do not account for slacks in the efficiency score. If DEA is used as a method for the evaluation of sales reps in practice it must be able to distinguish unmistakably between efficient and inefficient sales reps. This requirement is not provided by the CCR model because the calculated efficiency scores imply weak and strong efficient units. These units are not distinguished further and are all called efficient, despite the fact that some units still have slack values for further improvement. Hence, based on the CCR model, it is not possible to establish a fair compensation scheme.

A further obstacle is the fact that the CCR model implies the assumption of constant returns to scale which is questionable. So far output was maximized for given inputs. This seems to be logical for sales force evaluation because the task is to sell as much as possible. The problem with the CCR model is that DEA calculates unrealistically high output goals for some sales reps because the output side is expanded radially for given input levels until an efficient relationship between inputs and outputs is reached. For an example Table 4.1.2-7 is considered.

SR 53	Current Value	Target Value	Maximum from base data
TR	96%	160%	131%
CI	36%	55%	43%
SOM	36%	55%	43%

Table 4.1.2-7: Maximum projection and maximum value achieved

The table depicts current and target values for SR 53 for different CCR DEA versions. SR 53 is picked as an example because the calculated target values are the highest. The column "Maximum from base data" gives the maximum values from the base data (see appendix B) achieved by sales reps in the fourth quarter 2006. The question that arises is, whether or not it is realistic for a sales rep to achieve a target realization of 160% or a share of market of 55% if the best values from the base data for the fourth quarter 2006 accounted to 131% TR and 43% SOM? After consulting the pharmaceutical company the author suggests that reaching these high target values, as calculated by the CCR versions, is not possible.

The reason for the high output targets are the relative high input values of SR 53 (F: 93%, CCD: 378, CCP: 147, F/T: 86%). The output orientated DEA calculates outputs for *given inputs* and therefore assumes that SR 53 can transform all the inputs into outputs with the same marginal return on effort as the benchmark partners of SR 53 do. This is due to the underlying assumption of constant returns to scale of the CCR model which obviously does not hold.

Figure 4.1.2-2 clarifies this fact graphically in the single output (TR) single input (CCD) space. With the VRS assumption the projected output level is as high as P^{VRS} and with the CRS assumption as high as P^{CRS}. Due to the fact that the distance between the two output projections of SR 53 (and of a lot of other sales reps in the CCR case) is fairly big, it seems to be wise to stick to the VRS assumption.

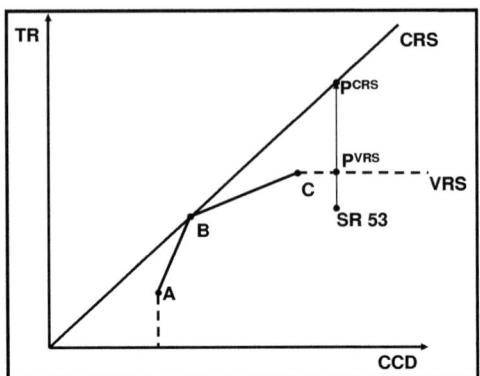

Figure 4.1.2-2: Difference in BCC and CCR output projection

The problem with an overestimation of projected outputs when using the CCR model does not occur in models with variable returns to scale.

In the next chapter the BCC model will be introduced to point out the impact on the results when a change to the DEA model has been made.

4.2 Results of the BCC model

As explained in chapter 4.1 DEA can be applied to the case of variable returns to scale as well. For sales force evaluation the case of variable returns to scale is worth thinking of. Intuitively changes in the input structure of a sales rep do not result into proportional output changes. Henceforth it is worth looking at a DEA model with variable returns to scale by applying the standard BCC model to the evaluation of the sales force. Similar to chapter 4.1 the output orientated BCC model will be applied to the five different input and output settings.

4.2.1 DEA setting with four inputs and two outputs (F, CCD, CCP, F/T - Q, CI)

Using F, CCD, CCP, F/T as inputs and Q and CI as outputs the DEA BCC model is run.

The Efficiency Gap

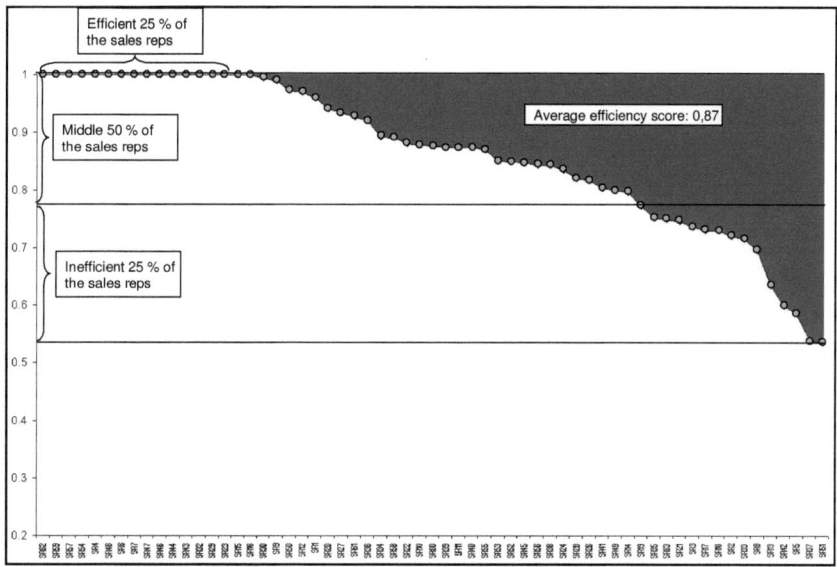

Figure 4.2.1-1: The efficiency gap for the BCC model version 1

Figure 4.2.1-1 displays the efficiency gap for the first version of the BCC model. The presented efficiency scores do not include slacks. The efficiency scores of the sample range between 0.53 and 1. The average efficiency score of the sample in this setting is 0.87. Compared with the CCR version in chapter 4.1 the average efficiency score is 0.03 points higher. This is due to the fact that the BCC version of DEA covers the data with a tighter efficiency frontier and therefore most of the inefficient DMUs lie closer to the frontier which results into higher efficiency scores.

Version 1	Average BCC Efficiency	Average CCR Efficiency
Efficient 25%	100%	100%
Middle 50%	89%	82%
Inefficient 25%	68%	64%

Table 4.2.1-1: Results of the BCC and CCR model

This fact becomes additionally clear when comparing the average efficiency scores for the different groups depicted in Table 4.2.1-1. The efficiency scores for the BCC version are all higher than for the CCR version. The highest difference regarding the average efficiency score between the two models is detected in the middle class and accounts to 7%. For the BCC setting the efficient 25 % achieve an average efficiency score of 100%, the middle group 89% and the inefficient 25% an average score of 68%.

A closer look at the input and output characteristics displayed in Table 4.2.1-2 of the groups reveals that several statistically significant ($p \leq 5\%$) characteristics occur.

➢ The mean ranks of the input F between the efficiency groups do not differ significantly.

➢ There is no significant difference in the mean ranks of CCD between the groups in this setting. This means that CCD cannot be taken as explanation for differences in efficiency realization among the groups *in this setting*.

Input/Output	Group	Group Average	Mean rank	z-value	doublesided p-value
Frequency	efficient 25%	0.75	18.90	-1.5900	0.1118
	middle 50%	0.84	25.70		
	efficient 25%	0.75	14.40	-0.6800	0.4965
	inefficient 25%	0.81	16.60		
	middle 50%	0.84	25.10	1.1200	0.2627
	inefficient 25%	0.81	20.30		
CCD	efficient 25%	207	18.30	-1.8200	0.0688
	middle 50%	231	26.00		
	efficient 25%	207	15.20	-0.1700	0.8650
	inefficient 25%	215	15.80		
	middle 50%	231	25.70	1.5600	0.1188
	inefficient 25%	215	19.00		
CCP	efficient 25%	90	18.40	-1.7700	0.0767
	middle 50%	107	26.00		
	efficient 25%	90	13.40	-1.3100	0.1902
	inefficient 25%	102	17.60		
	middle 50%	107	24.10	0.4500	0.6527
	inefficient 25%	102	22.20		
F/T	efficient 25%	0.70	15.40	-2.8500	0.0044
	middle 50%	0.83	27.40		
	efficient 25%	0.70	11.30	-2.5700	0.0102
	inefficient 25%	0.83	19.70		
	middle 50%	0.83	23.90	0.2600	0.7949
	inefficient 25%	0.83	22.70		
Q	efficient 25%	6.35	21.10	0.8400	0.4009
	middle 50%	6.59	24.70		
	efficient 25%	6.35	20.10	-2.8200	0.0048
	inefficient 25%	4.87	10.90		
	middle 50%	6.59	28.40	3.5600	0.0004
	inefficient 25%	4.87	13.30		
CI	efficient 25%	0.36	26.90	-1.1800	0.2380
	middle 50%	0.34	21.90		
	efficient 25%	0.36	22.30	4.2100	<.0001
	inefficient 25%	0.26	8.70		
	middle 50%	0.34	30.20	4.8900	<.0001
	inefficient 25%	0.26	9.60		

Table 4.2.1-2: Differences between the efficiency groups regarding the input and output dimensions

- ➤ The mean ranks of the input CCP do not differ significantly between the groups and therefore cannot be relied on as argument for different efficiency measures.

- ➤ The input F/T is characterized by significant differences between the three groups. Therefore the efficient group is better than the other two groups in turning the fixed doctor relations into output. Hence the input F/T can explain differences in the efficiency scores between the groups.

- ➤ The output Q differs significantly between the inefficient 25% compared with the top and the middle group. Therefore this output is detected as one reason for the bad average efficiency score of the inefficient 25%. Hence the output Q is an important characteristic for distinguishing inefficient from efficient sales reps.

- ➤ The way the different groups cope with their competitors differs very significantly between the inefficient 25% compared with the top and the middle group. Another significant source of inefficiency considering the average efficiency score of the low group therefore stems from bad performance in the output category CI.

The results are similar to chapter 4.1.1 but do differ slightly due to the assumptions of VRS. Furthermore the number of efficient sales reps increased as result of the VRS assumption.

In case all of the sales reps would work efficiently in this DEA setting, target values displayed in Table 4.2.1-3 could be reached. Compared to the corresponding chapter 4.1.1 the increases on the output side are not as dramatic. The output Q only increases by 18% instead of 26% and the corresponding market share increases by 3% instead of nearly 6%. However the decreases on the input side are greater for every category than in chapter4.1.1.

Input/Output	Current Value	Target Value	Delta %
ØF	81%	80%	-1%
CCD	13517	13070	-3%
CCP	6245	5243	-16%
ØF/T	80%	76%	-4%
Q	373	440	18%
SOM	32%	35%	3%

Table 4.2.1-3: Optimal input and output projection for the BCC DEA model version 1

This finding stems from the fact that the efficiency frontier is drawn tighter around the data and therefore the possible space which reports slacks increases. As mentioned in previous chapters, once again the input CCP implies the biggest improvement potential.

Benchmarking of individual sales reps

Corresponding to the CCR section sales reps 4, 28 and 42 are used to demonstrate the impact of changes in the DEA arrangement on the individual results.

The results for sales rep 4 are displayed in Figure 4.2.1-2. Because sales rep 4 is efficient in version 1 with CRS this sales rep must be efficient under VRS as well. Therefore the efficient result is not unexpected. Both, current and projected values of SR 4´s inputs and outputs are the same and therefore SR 4 is not only weak efficient (radial efficient, but with slacks) but also strong efficient in the sense of Pareto-Koopmans-Efficiency (no slacks present). SR4 is benchmark partner for 16 inefficient sales reps and with the impact factor of 5.14 this sales rep ranks fourth with respect to the importance as mentor to improve inefficient colleagues.

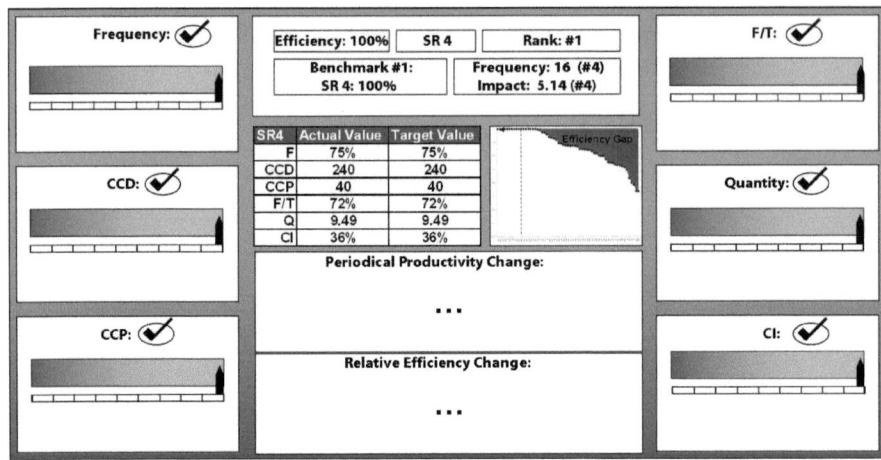

Figure 4.2.1-2: KPI Cockpit for SR4

Figure 4.2.1-3 presents the results for SR 28. With a score of 82% SR 28 is inefficient and could expand its outputs radially by 22% without changing inputs except for the input CCP, indicating that the quality of CCP should increase to reach the efficiency frontier. Differing from the corresponding CCR version, SR 28 has a slack of 3.5% in the input CCP which quantifies the extent of the necessary adjustment process in the input CCP.

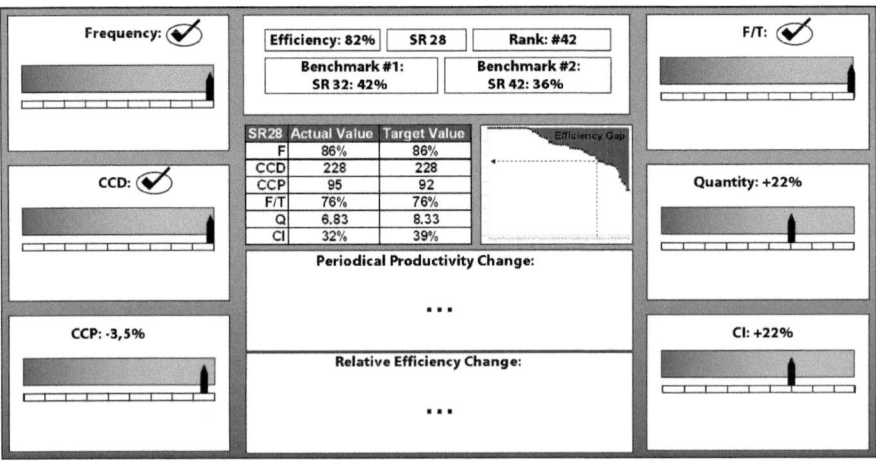

Figure 4.2.1-3: KPI Cockpit for SR28

As Figure 4.2.1-4 displays SR 42 reached an efficiency score of 59% and is ranked #58. The two most important benchmarks for SR 42 are SR 44 with 63% and SR 6 with 33%. SR 42 has an input slack of 10% in the input frequency and on the output side major increases should be undertaken to reach the efficiency frontier. In addition to expanding both outputs radial by 66%, SR 42 should expand Q by the output slack of 181%. Once again the DEA model detects high improvement potential for SR 42 and therefore SR 42 should be reevaluated.

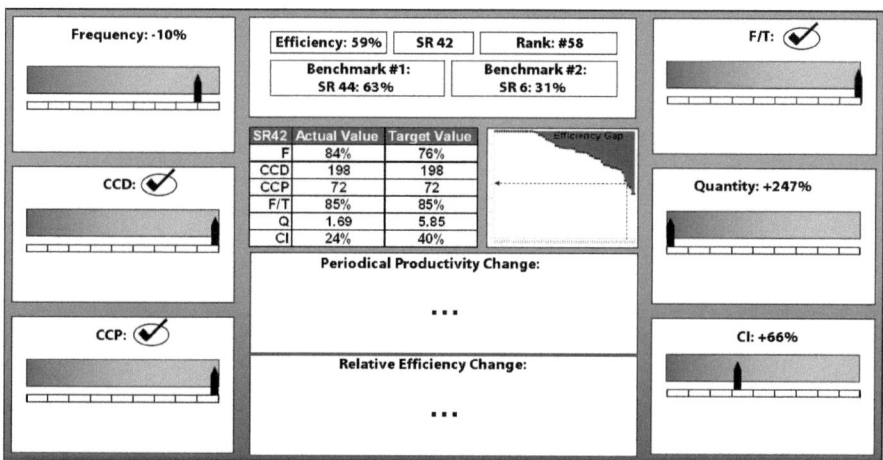

Figure 4.2.1-4: KPI Cockpit for SR42

4.2.2 Summary of the BCC DEA model

Section 4.2 presented results for five different BCC DEA versions. In this section the main results of the section 4.2 are summarized. Figure 4.2.2-1 depicts the efficiency gaps for all of the different DEA settings.

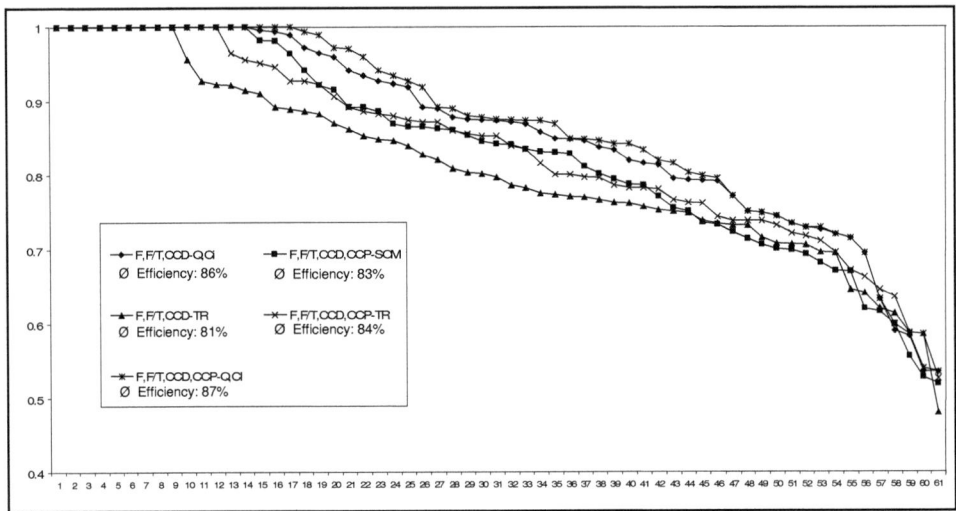

Figure 4.2.2-1: Summary of the efficiency gap for the BCC DEA versions

It is obvious that the four dimensional setting with the F, F/T and CCD as inputs and TR as output (line with triangles) results into the strictest efficiency measure because the triangle line is the lowest and therefore the average efficiency score is the lowest as well (81%).
As in chapter 4.1.2 the graphs above reveal the tendency that a rising amount of inputs and outputs for a given number of DMUs results into increasing average efficiency scores. The highest average efficiency score of 87% (line with stars) is reached by the six dimensional setting with F, F/T, CCD, CCP as inputs and Q and CI as outputs.

The summaries for the sales reps 4, 28 and 42 are presented in the tables below. The percentage values in the input and output lines are the percentage decreases (for inputs) and increases (for outputs) referring to the status quo. The benchmark lines display the impact of the different efficient SRs as mentoring partner for the evaluated sales rep (SR4, 28, 42) in the specific setting. The columns show the different DEA settings. The last line depicts the efficiency score of the evaluated sales rep in each of the DEA variants.

Sales Reps 4		(1) F,F/T,CCD,CCP-Q,CI	(2) F,F/T,CCD-Q,CI	(3) F,F/T,CCD,CCP-SOM	(4) F,F/T,CCD,CCP-TR	(5) F,F/T,CCD-TR
Inputs	F	0.00%	0.00%	0.00%	0.00%	0.00%
	CCD	0.00%	0.00%	0.00%	0.00%	-7.06%
	CCP	0.00%	~	0.00%	~	~
	F/T	0.00%	0.00%	0.00%	0.00%	0.00%
Outputs	Q	0.00%	0.00%	~	0.00%	~
	CI	0.00%	0.00%	~	0.00%	~
	TR	~	~	0.00%	~	14.87%
	SOM	~	~	~	~	~
Benchmarks	SR6	~	~	~	~	0.29
	SR30	~	~	~	~	0.53
	SR54	~	~	~	~	0.17
Efficiency		100%	100%	100%	100%	87%

Table 4.2.2-1: Summary of SR4 for the different BCC DEA versions

Sales rep 4 in Table 4.2.2-1 is inefficient only in the setting (5) with F, F/T, CCD as inputs and TR as output. Therefore only in this setting benchmark partners are assigned to SR 4 and an output expansion of 14.87% is calculated. Hence, when CCP is included SR4 achieves higher efficiency scores which indicate that CCP is contributing positively to the performance of SR4. In the BCC model the benchmark weights (sum of λ) add up to one and henceforth they can be interpreted as percentage impact of an efficient sales rep as mentor for inefficient sales rep. When the sum of λ is bounded to unity (see chapter 2.4) SR4 has an input slack in version 5.

SR 28 is inefficient in every BCC DEA version. The efficiency scores of SR 28 range between 76% (5) and 82% (1). SR 28 has got slacks on the input side in every version. Compared with the other versions, SR 28 faces high slacks in the input F/T in version (4) and (2). The reason for the increased reductions in the input side is due to the BCC efficiency frontier which covers the data closer and hence opens more room for slacks. In all BCC versions the optimal output can be reached by radial expansion.

Table 4.2.2-2 displays that SR 30 in version (5), SR 46 and SR 32 in version (1), SR 29 in version (4) and SR 54 in version (5) and (4) are the most important benchmarks for the evaluation for SR 28 because they have the biggest impact on the evaluation of the inefficiency of SR 28.

SR28		(1) F,F/T,CCD,CCP-Q,CI	(2) F,F/T,CCD-Q,CI	(3) F,F/T,CCD,CCP-SOM	(4) F,F/T,CCD,CCP-TR	(5) F,F/T,CCD-TR
Inputs	F	0.00%	0.00%	-2.28%	-4.40%	0.00%
	CCD	0.00%	0.00%	0.00%	0.00%	-2.72%
	CCP	-3.51%	~	0.00%	0.00%	~
	F/T	0.00%	-21.26%	0.00%	-22.28%	0.00%
Outputs	Q	21.99%	21.99%	~	~	~
	CI	21.99%	21.99%	~	~	~
	TR	~	~	~	24.91%	31.92%
	SOM	~	~	27.01%	~	~
Benchmarks	SR6	~	~	0.15	~	~
	SR 15	~	~	0.71	~	~
	SR16	0.14	~	~	~	~
	SR32	0.42	~	~	~	~
	SR 29	~	1.00	~	~	~
	SR30	~	~	~	0.24	0.78
	SR43	~	~	~	~	~
	SR44	0.01	~	~	~	~
	SR 46	0.42	~	0.03	~	~
	SR47	~	~	~	~	~
	SR48	~	~	~	~	~
	SR54	~	~	~	0.20	0.22
	SR59	~	~	~	0.57	~
	SR62	0.01	~	0.11	~	~
Efficiency		82%	82%	79%	80%	76%

Table 4.2.2-2: Summary of SR28 for the different BCC DEA versions

Table 4.2.2-3 presents the summary for SR 42. The efficiency scores of SR 42 range between 59% in version (2) and 66% in version (4). Similar to the CCR version it is interesting to mention that the worst efficiency score occurs in version (2). SR 28 had the worst efficiency score in version (5). Hence SR 42 is more efficient when evaluated with TR and SR28 is more efficient when evaluated with Q and CI as outputs. Thus, if Q and CI are included as outputs (version 2) SR 42 falls back compared to SR 28.

SR 42 has input slacks in all versions except in version (2). The slacks occur in the inputs F/T and F.

On the output side there are huge increases necessary to reach an efficient status. The amount of insulin sold should be expanded by about 240% in version (1) and (2). In addition, the way SR 42 faces competition has to be changed significantly compared to the efficient

SRs. Turning the attention to version (3), the market share has to be increased by 67% on the basis of the status quo. This goes in line with the vast increase of Q in (1) and (2). In addition SR 42 is far below the optimal target realization as indicated by the results of versions (5) and (4). The main benchmark partners for SR 42 are SR 4, SR 43 and SR 44.

SR 42		(1) F,F/T,CCD,CCP-Q,CI	(2) F,F/T,CCD-Q,CI	(3) F,F/T,CCD,CCP-SOM	(4) F,F/T,CCD,CCP-TR	(5) F,F/T,CCD-TR
Inputs	F	-9.66%	0.00%	-9.66%	-4.40%	0.00%
	CCD	0.00%	0.00%	0.00%	0.00%	0.00%
	CCP	0.00%	~	0.00%	0.00%	~
	F/T	0.00%	0.00%	0.00%	-22.28%	-8.43%
Outputs	Q	247.00%	239.72%	~	~	~
	CI	66.85%	69.50%	~	~	~
	TR	~	~	~	24.91%	63.09%
	SOM	~	~	66.85%	~	~
Benchmarks	SR4	0.04	~	0.04	0.13	~
	SR6	0.31	~	0.31	~	~
	SR30	~	~	~	~	0.52
	SR43	~	~	~	0.09	0.29
	SR44	0.63	0.66	0.63	~	~
	SR46	~	0.08	~	~	~
	SR47	0.02	~	0.02	~	~
	SR48	~	0.15	~	~	~
	SR54	~	~	~	0.66	0.18
	SR59	~	0.08	~	0.11	~
	SR62	~	~	0.10	~	~
Efficiency		60%	59%	60%	66%	61%

Table 4.2.2-3: Summary of SR42 for the different BCC DEA versions

Table 4.2.2-4 displays the frequencies of efficient sales reps in the benchmark sets of inefficient sales reps for the five DEA versions. Sales reps that are only mentioned one time are benchmarks to themselves. SR 54 is mentioned 100 times followed by SR30 with 90 times mentioned. SR 43 is mentioned in every DEA variant as benchmark partner which indicates that this sales rep is in the efficient group in each variant. SR 6 is not mentioned as frequently as SR 43 but belongs to the efficient group in every version. SR 15 is mentioned 5 times and is only efficient in version (1) and (3). SR 54 and 30 seem to have their advantages in the measure target realization. SR 32 for instance is only efficient when looking at the amount of insulin sold and the CI as output.

Sales Reps	(1) F,F/T,CCD,CCP-Q,CI	(2) F,F/T,CCD-Q,CI	(3) F,F/T,CCD,CCP-SOM	(4) F,F/T,CCD,CCP-TR	(5) F,F/T,CCD-TR	Sum
SR4	16	6	7	6	0	35
SR6	10	7	26	4	8	55
SR7	1	1	0	0	0	2
SR15	1	0	4	0	0	5
SR16	14	18	0	0	0	32
SR23	3	4	3	2	5	17
SR29	1	1	4	2	5	13
SR30	0	0	0	41	49	90
SR32	30	33	0	0	0	63
SR43	11	12	13	17	24	77
SR44	24	24	32	0	0	80
SR46	28	31	32	0	0	91
SR47	1	0	4	1	0	6
SR48	5	5	12	1	1	24
SR54	6	6	1	44	43	100
SR57	1	0	1	1	0	3
SR59	1	1	2	30	3	37
SR62	14	20	22	3	5	64
Sum	167	169	163	152	143	794

Table 4.2.2-4: Frequencies of efficient sales reps in the benchmark sets of inefficient sales reps

Table 4.2.2-5 depicts the cumulated benchmark weights of an efficient sales rep for each DEA version. If the focus is on the summed up benchmark weights, SR 30 is the most important and has a very high impact as mentor in the two efficient cases with TR as output. Interestingly, SR 46 is, despite the fact that SR 46 is only efficient in version (1), (2) and (3) the second important. This indicates that SR46 is very good in the output categories Q and CI. The least important as mentor is SR 15 which goes hand in hand with the finding of the table above

Table 4.2.2-6 summarizes the output projections of each DEA version transformed into market share and amount of insulin sold (in MMU). The projected amount of Q sold varies between 440 MMU (+18%) and 477 MMU (+28%) depending on the DEA version applied. The corresponding market share projections vary between 35.15% (+3.36 % points) and 38.1% (+6.31% points).

Sales Reps	(1)F,F/T,CCD,CCP-Q,CI	(2) F,F/T,CCD-Q,CI	(3) F,F/T,CCD,CCP-SOM	(4) F,F/T,CCD,CCP-TR	(5) F,F/T,CCD-TR	Sum
SR4	5.14	3.13	2.23	2.07	0.00	12.56
SR6	2.83	2.25	7.48	2.12	2.69	17.37
SR 7	1.00	1.00	0.00	0.00	0.00	2.00
SR15	1.00	0.00	2.48	0.00	0.00	3.48
SR16	4.94	6.19	0.00	0.00	0.00	11.13
SR23	1.88	2.42	1.62	1.56	2.36	9.84
SR29	1.53	1.53	1.52	1.70	1.92	8.22
SR30	0.00	0.00	0.00	16.69	30.95	47.64
SR32	9.79	11.11	0.00	0.00	0.00	20.90
SR43	2.69	2.37	3.56	4.59	5.54	18.76
SR44	6.69	6.86	12.19	0.00	0.00	25.73
SR46	11.57	12.74	12.65	0.00	0.00	36.95
SR47	1.02	0.00	1.81	1.00	0.00	3.82
SR48	2.02	1.59	4.24	1.60	1.60	11.04
SR54	2.47	2.47	1.00	13.98	11.28	31.19
SR57	1.00	0.00	1.00	1.00	0.00	3.00
SR59	1.21	1.21	1.11	13.53	1.90	18.96
SR62	4.23	6.14	8.13	1.11	2.75	22.35
Sum	61.00	61.00	61.00	61.00	61.00	305.00

Table 4.2.2-5: Impact factors of the efficient sales reps as benchmark for the sample

Therefore the BCC version of DEA indicates a potential market share increase to at least 35.15% for the fourth quarter 2006 by making the inefficient sales reps work as well as the efficient ones in the sample.

BCC DEA Version	Unit	Actual Value	Target Value	Delta
F,F/T,CCD,CCP-Q,CI	Q	372.70	440.00	18.06%
	SOM	31.79%	35.15%	3.36%
F,F/T,CCD-Q,CI	Q	373	443	18.86%
	SOM	31%	35%	4.01%
F,F/T,CCD,CCP-TR	Q	372.70	463.00	24.23%
	SOM	31.79%	36.99%	5.19%
F,F/T,CCD-TR	Q	372.70	477.00	27.98%
	SOM	31.79%	38.10%	6.31%
F,F/T,CCD,CCP-SOM	Q	372.70	453.00	21.55%
	SOM	31.79%	36.19%	4.39%

Table 4.2.2-6: Optimal output projections for the five BCC DEA versions

Critical annotations on the BCC model

Regarding the fact that the efficiency scores of the BCC model imply weak and strong efficient units this DEA model has the same shortcomings regarding practical application as the CCR model has. Due to ambiguous efficiency score no clear ranking can be established, which questions the possibility for a fair compensation of sales rep based on the efficiency score.

Chapter 4.2 presented an overview over possible DEA settings, evaluated using the output orientated BCC method. In the next chapter the SBM model will be presented and the reasons why the SBM model suits sales evaluation better than the CCR and BCC model will be stated.

4.3 Results of the inter-temporal, non orientated SBM model with VRS

The preceding chapters 4.1 and 4.2 focused on an output orientated utilization of the CCR and BCC DEA model calculated for the fourth quarter of 2006. Despite the fact that the CCR and BCC models calculate usable results several severe shortcomings have to be considered, which are due to the radial efficiency measures of the models, the constant returns to scale assumption of the CCR model, the output orientation and the static nature of the models (focus only on the fourth quarter 2006).

> The main shortcoming of the CCR and BCC efficiency scores is that they do not account for the slack values (see Tone 2001). As described above one has to distinguish weak from strong efficient sales reps. Weak efficient sales reps have been assigned efficient DEA scores but they still have slacks. Strong efficient sales reps have not got slacks. Both strong and weak efficient sales reps achieve the same efficiency score of one. The question arising is how to handle the slack values? Of course a weak efficient sales rep cannot be as efficient as strong efficient sales reps are. Henceforth all units with slacks should be brought into a rank order. One way of creating a rank order that accounts for slacks would be to put bounds on the shadow prices (see Ray 2004), which would deflate the DEA score. Beside others, the problem is that the chosen weights would be subjective and would not have been calculated endogenously by the optimization problem. This is a major shortcoming of the radial models which ruins every serious attempt to establish a fair compensation system for sales reps. Therefore a model for the DEA calculation has to be chosen that incorporates slack values into the efficiency score. The SBM model solves the problem because it accounts for slacks and calculates comparable efficiency scores ranging between 0 and 1.

In addition to the problems with the overestimation of *realistic* optimal outputs in the CCR model (see summary of CCR model, chapter 4.1.2) due to the constant return to scale assumption, the efficiency scores of both DEA models deployed so far (CCR and BCC) neglect optimization opportunities on the input side because of their output orientation. To reveal optimization possibilities that influence the efficiency score from the input side as well a non orientated calculation of efficiency scores should be utilized to find an optimal balance between inputs and outputs. From a practical point of view this proposition has the following legitimation: If a sales rep has a lot of optimization potential on the input side this fact indicates that this sales rep is working under low quality of inputs, which will shows up in low shadow prices. The pharmaceutical company is very interested in increasing both, on the one hand side the sales volume and on the other hand side the quality of operations. Thus, both sides should be optimized, the input and output side.

➢ A further limitation of the models presented so far is that they only focus on the fourth quarter 2006. This may result into misleading conclusions for the sales force evaluation due to wrong benchmarks. The main problem is that outliers within a time period may influence the results negatively. For instance it can occure that sales rep X has reached an efficient status in one period, because of specific market condition for example, but was very inefficient in the other periods. In a case like that it is not sensible to use sales rep X as mentor for others, because it is not sure yet if the good performance in the last time period of SR X is just a matter of chance or if it is a long term upswing. Henceforth it is important to evaluate the sales force over time. This can be achieved by calculating efficiency values for every single period to track the efficiency development of a sales rep. But still, only concentrating on relative efficiency measures may be not enough. It is important to look at productivity developments as well. The case may come about where the overall productivity of the evaluated sales force decreases along with the productivity of the sales rep under consideration. Despite the productivity decrease the relative efficiency of the evaluated sales rep may increase because the productivity decrease of the sales rep under evaluation was not as severe as the overall decrease of the sales force. For every company a case as described above is unfavourable and revealing the sources of productivity decrease can be crucial. Therefore, the relative efficiency measure on its own does not provide enough information to rely on for an in depth sales force analysis. What the sales management needs is the Malmquist Productivity Index (MPI) as described in chapter two, which is able to track productivity developments over time and, therefore, controls for, whether increases in relative efficiency (indicated by the catch up process) are accompanied by increases in overall productivity (indicated by the frontier shift).

In addition to the already presented ranking of inefficient units DEA provides a method for ranking the efficient units as well. This concept was not applied up to know to keep the present analysis lean. However, in the following pages the concept of super efficiency will be addressed but *only* for ranking the efficient sales reps and for the calculation of the MPI[16]. From a managerial point of view a ranking of the efficient units is essential. In case several sales reps are efficient, there still may be differences in how far a specific sales rep "drags out" the efficiency frontier (see chapter 2.4.4). The more important a sales rep is in forming the efficiency frontier, the higher the super-efficiency rank is and the higher the rewarded compensation may be.

Considering the points mentioned above, the model of choice is the non orientated super slack based measurement model with variable returns to scale (NO-(Super)-SBM-V) and a non radial MPI with variable returns to scale. This model, which accounts for all shortcomings of the BCC and CCR models named above, will be used in the second, inter temporal empirical part of this thesis to evaluate the sales force.

Similar to the foregoing chapters the SBM model *will be presented in five different input and output arrangements*. In contrast to chapter 4.1.2, the most contributing factor to efficiency will not be uncovered by checking for significant differences in the group averages of the inputs and outputs. Instead, the input and output multipliers directly resulting from the SBM calculation will be used to reveal sources of efficiency. These multipliers depict the effect of a marginal input output change on the efficiency score and therefore quantify the factor productivity of a sales rep in a dimension. Unfortunately this method was not applicable to the CCR and BCC models because of the existence of slacks. In case a DMU has a slack in an input or output, it is wasting resources and therefore, corresponding with the duality theory, the specific multiplier is zero. As explained in the methodical part, the SBM model overcomes this problem due to the inclusion of slacks and therefore the problem of zero multipliers does

---

[16] The MPI using the super efficiency concept is applied due to the fact that infeasible solutions which would occur using the MPI based on the NO-SBM-V are avoided

not exist (see appendix B). Hence a comparison of multipliers in the SBM model between the groups is possible.

The concept of the efficiency gap is the same as in the previous chapters but despite the calculation of super efficiency scores the scores for the computation of the efficiency gap will be bounded to one. The reason for this is that the main interest lies in the visualisation and calculation of the prevailing inefficiencies. The super efficiency score will be ranked and commented separately.

In addition, inter-temporal aspects for each of the five variants will be highlighted. In detail the average efficiency development and the median MPI of the total sample is presented for each time period. For the calculation of the average efficiency score of the sample presented with the efficiency gap, the author will stick to the classical approach with maximum efficiency scores of one. The advantage of such procedure is that no super efficiency score will artificially increase the average efficiency.

Moreover, the individual sales reps inter-temporal development regarding the relative efficiency score and the MPI will be assessed to check for whether or not the results of the analysis of the fourth quarter 2006 are an exception or the rule.

The fact that the BCC model assumes VRS but does not account for slacks disqualifies it for the further usage in this dissertation. Nevertheless, to continue with the research a model with variable returns to scale which incorporates slacks in the calculation of efficiency measures should be applied. Hence, in this section 4.3 the non orientated (Super) SBM model with variable returns to scale will be applied for the sales force evaluation.

4.3.1 SBM Model Version 1 (F, CCD, CCP, F/T, Q, CI)

In this section the SBM version presented implies F, CCD, CCP, F/T as inputs and Q and CI as outputs.

The Efficiency Gap

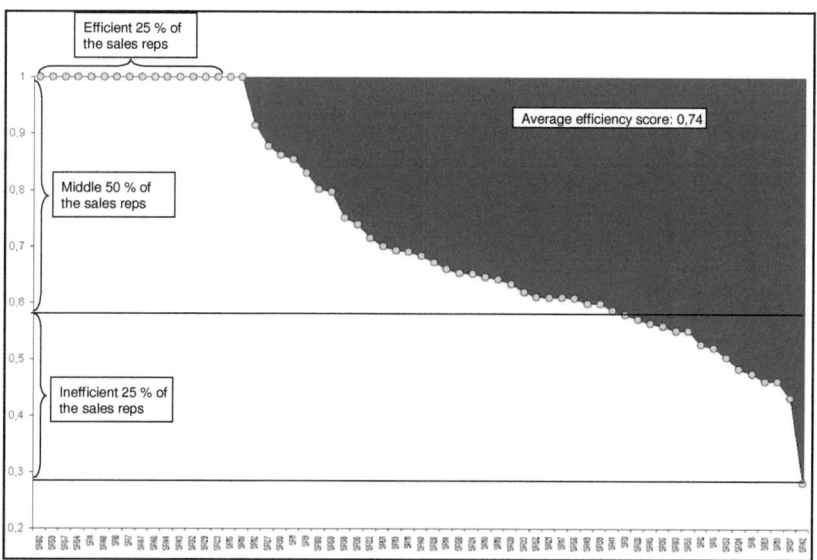

Figure 4.3.1-1: Illustration of the Efficiency Gap and of the three efficiency groups

Figure 4.3.1-1 displays the efficiency gap for the first version of the SBM model. In contrast to the CCR and BCC model the graphical presentation of the efficiency gap accounts for slacks. The efficiency scores of the sample range between 0.28 and 1. The average efficiency score of the sample in this setting is 0.74. Compared with the CCR version in chapter 4.1.1 and the BCC version in chapter 4.2.1 the average efficiency score is 0.07 lower and 0.13 points lower for the latter. This is mainly due to the fact that the SBM version of DEA includes slacks in the calculation of the efficiency scores and therefore all efficient sales reps are Pareto-Koopmans-Efficient.

F,CCD,CCP,F/T - Q,CI Group	Average SBM-NO-V Efficiency	Average BCC-O Efficiency	Average CCR-O Efficiency
Efficient 25%	100%	100%	100%
Middle 50%	76%	89%	82%
Inefficient 25%	52%	68%	64%

Table 4.3.1-1: Comparison of average efficiency scores

Table 4.3.1-1 compares the average efficiency scores of the groups in the SBM version with the average scores of the BCC and CCR versions. The scores of the middle and inefficient 25% in the SBM version are the lowest ones attained[17]. The top groups in all versions attain an efficiency score of 100%.

To discover differences between the three efficiency groups regarding the input and output multipliers the Mann-Whitney-U Test is applied, because the assumption of a normal distribution within the groups does not hold. Table 4.3.1-2 reveals the differences in the inputs and outputs. A statistically significant difference can be assured at a level of $p \leq 5\%$.

The first column shows the input and output categories. The second displays the groups that are compared to each other. The third column presents the average group multipliers of the primal problem. These average multipliers can also be interpreted as the average virtual prices (see chapter two) for one unit of input or output in the specific groups. The higher the price is for a particular input in a group compared to the other groups is, the more efficient a group uses this input.

The fourth column depicts the mean rank. For the Mann-Whitney-U Test the data of the two groups compared is ranked beginning with the lowest and ending with the highest value. Therefore a lower mean rank reveals lower virtual weights of the analyzed dimension and a higher mean rank indicates higher virtual weights.

Column five and six show the test statistic z and the corresponding double sided p-value respectively. The results of Table 4.3.1-2 can be interpreted the following way:

---

[17] The reason for this finding may be multiple: at first the SBM model used includes slacks and is non-orientated. These two facts make it a sharper efficiency measure than the output orientated BCC model. In this case the non-orientated SBM model with VRS is an even sharper efficiency measure than the CCR model which has CRS. If the effect on the efficiency scores of the non-orientation and the inclusion of slacks is very low and the effect of the scale assumption on the efficiency scores very high, the CCR model may be a sharper efficiency measure than the NO-SBM-V model is and the results of Table 4.3.1-1 between the CCR and SBM model may differ.

- The efficient 25 % use the input frequency significantly more efficient than the middle and the inefficient group. With an average multiplier of 1.3 the virtual price for the input frequency is more than three times higher in the top group than in the middle group. The same result holds for the difference between the top group and the inefficient 25%. The Mann-Whitney-U Test comes to a similar conclusion. The higher mean ranks of the efficient 25% regarding the input frequency indicate a more efficient use of this input by these sales reps compared to the other sales reps. The difference between the middle and the lower group is not significant and can be neglected.

- Amazingly there is no significantly difference in the mean ranks of CCD between the groups in this setting. This means that CCD can not be taken as explanation for differences in efficiency realization among the groups *in this setting*. This result highlights that *in this setting* there is a similar factor productivity between the quartiles.

- The mean ranks of the input CCP differ significant between the efficient and middle group and between the efficient and inefficient group. This finding gives the information that the virtual price for one call to a pharmacy is higher in the top group than in the other two groups which in turn leads to the conclusion that the top group uses the input CCP most efficiently. The difference between the middle group and the inefficient 25% is not significant.

- The input F/T is characterized by very significant differences between the three groups. The efficient group has a higher mean rank for a F/T unit than in the other two groups. This means that the leverage effect on efficiency of the input fixed doctor relations in the efficient group is higher compared to the other groups. The difference between the middle and the low group is not significant.

- For the output Q the top group reaches a significantly higher average virtual price per unit than the other groups. For the middle group the average virtual price is lower than that of the top group and higher than the one of the low group. Hence, regarding the output Q clear distinctions between the three groups can be made considering the relationship of the virtual price and the achieved efficiency score.

➢ The competition index was added to this setting to adjust for inhomogeneous market deployments and it is used for evaluating the competitiveness of a salesman. Part of the definition of the competition index is that the CI cannot be set equal with the market share because of differing optimal projection values between Q and CI. However the projections of Q and CI have the same tendency and henceforth propositions like "SR X should increase his competitiveness" can be made. The top group has the highest mean rank for CI followed by the middle group. The inefficient 25% are assigned the lowest mean rank. This fact leads to the conclusion that higher efficiency comes along with higher competitiveness.

There is one important point to mention: due to the fact that the inputs and outputs consist of both absolute and relative numbers caution is demanded when interpreting the importance of an input or output for the production with the help of the multipliers. Per definition the multipliers (virtual costs) are the LaGrange-Multipliers and quantify the effect on the objective function when one of the constraints is changed. For Table 4.3.1-3 this would mean that the virtual cost for CCD would change by 0,0112 if CCD would be changed by one unit for the efficient 25%. The same interpretation is valid for the input F. If F is changed by one unit, the virtual cost for the input F would change by 1.3 for the efficient group. **_BUT_** increasing (for example) F by one unit worth 1.3 would mean increasing the input F by 100% points up to an average Frequency of 173%. This of course is not sensible because the multipliers can only be interpreted on the basis of *marginal changes*. For that reasoning the multipliers can only be compared within an input or output category for very small changes. To compare the importance of the different categories for the overall production process of a sales rep, the virtual worth of the dimension should be calculated, i.e. virtual price times the input or output data of a SR. Table 4.3.1-3 displays the average group data for the different categories weighted with the average multipliers which results into the virtual worth of a dimension.

Input/Output	Group	Group Average Weights	Mean Rank	z-value	doublesided p-value
Frequency	efficient 25%	1.3	29.3	2.02	0.0434
	middle 50%	0.4	20.7		
	efficient 25%	1.3	19.3	2.34	0.0193
	inefficient 25%	0.36	11.7		
	middle 50%	0.4	24.00	0.37	0.7114
	inefficient 25%	0.36	22.4		
CCD	efficient 25%	0.0112	27.6	1.43	0.1527
	middle 50%	0.0031	21.5		
	efficient 25%	0.0112	18.1	1.58	0.1141
	inefficient 25%	0.0026	12.9		
	middle 50%	0.0031	24.9	0.98	0.3271
	inefficient 25%	0.0026	20.7		
CCP	efficient 25%	0.0213	31.1	2.66	0.0078
	middle 50%	0.0026	19.8		
	efficient 25%	0.0213	20.4	3.03	0.0024
	inefficient 25%	0.0024	10.6		
	middle 50%	0.0026	25.5	1.45	0.1471
	inefficient 25%	0.0024	19.3		
F/T	efficient 25%	5.76	30.7	2.53	0.0114
	middle 50%	0.52	20.00		
	efficient 25%	5.76	19.8	2.68	0.0074
	inefficient 25%	0.34	11.2		
	middle 50%	0.52	23.4	-0.05	0.9601
	inefficient 25%	0.34	23.7		
Q	efficient 25%	0.15	37.1	4.76	<.0001
	middle 50%	0.07	16.9		
	efficient 25%	0.15	22.3	4.23	<.0001
	inefficient 25%	0.05	8.7		
	middle 50%	0.07	24.00	0.36	0.7188
	inefficient 25%	0.05	22.4		
CI	efficient 25%	6.65	34.7	3.94	0.0001
	middle 50%	2.22	18.1		
	efficient 25%	6.65	21.8	3.9	<.0001
	inefficient 25%	1.42	9.2		
	middle 50%	2.22	26.7	2.3	0.0214
	inefficient 25%	1.42	16.9		

Table 4.3.1-2: Relationship between average efficiency scores and input and output multipliers

The efficient group has the highest average virtual worth (input output data times the shadow price (same as virtual price)) in all categories which indicates that this group uses the inputs most efficiently in relation to outputs. Unfortunately, the virtual worth of some dimensions of the efficient 25% is very high compared to the inefficient groups. This is due to high virtual weights for some efficient sales reps in the data set due to a special transformation system from inputs to outputs.

Groups	F	CCD	CCP	F/T	Q	CI
efficient 25%	0,87	2,29	1,88	4,12	1,00	13,33
middle 50%	0,31	0,66	0,25	0,36	0,37	0,79
inefficient 25%	0,31	0,55	0,26	0,27	0,25	0,45

Table 4.3.1-3: Average virtual worth of the input or output category

The biggest improvement potential regarding efficiency is where the virtual worth of an input or output category is the lowest within the two inefficient groups. The reasoning behind this suggestion is that a low virtual worth of a dimension indicates an inefficient use of resources within that dimension. Henceforth, on the input side the CCP seems to have a big improvement potential and on the output side Q. Therefore, when cutting down CCP and increasing Q for the two inefficient groups, the virtual prices of both CCP and Q will rise. Rising virtual worth indicates a more efficient use/production of inputs/outputs.

Not only CCP and Q can be optimized, but also the other inputs and outputs, albeit CCP and Q have the biggest improvement potential. This finding goes in line with the following results of Table 4.3.1-4 which give an overview over current and optimal inputs and output values regarding the whole sample.

Table 4.3.1-4 presents the target values for the overall sales force in case all sales reps would attain an efficiency score of 100%.

Input/Output	Current Value	Target Value	Delta %
ØF	81%	77%	-4%
CCD	13517	13080	-3%
CCP	6245	4200	-33%
ØF/T	80%	72%	-8%
Q	373	504	35%
SOM	32%	40%	8%

Table 4.3.1-4: Comparison of current and optimal target values

The SBM setting calculates slack based measures instead of radial projected measures and therefore calculates non radial reductions or increases for the inputs and outputs. Similar to the CCR and BCC model the SBM model reveals the biggest efficiency reserves in the input CCP with an optimal overall value decreased by 33%. Compared to the CCR and BCC model the increase in the input Q is much higher and is calculated to be 35% higher in an efficient status. This amount of Q would result into a market share increase of 8%.

Inter-temporal aspects

Figure 4.3.1-2 presents the development of the average inputs and outputs over the twelve quarters from 2004 to 2006[18]. The average quantity of insulin sold per quarter increased sharply over the last three years. This indicates fast growing demand for insulin. However, despite increasing sales volume the market share declined.
The graphs depict that the two inputs Frequency and F/T stayed more or less constant. The input CCP has three peeks in q3 2004, q3 2005 and q3 2006.
The input CCD has got two peeks in q3 2004 and q3 2006 where the average CCD per sales rep are significantly higher than in the other quarters.

Considering Figure 4.3.1-2 the conclusion that the productivity followed an upward trend from year to year lies at hand. On the output side the strong increase in insulin sales overshadows the slow CI decrease. A closer look at the graphic leads to the assumption that the productivity decreased from q3 to q4 2004, from q2 to q3 2005 and from q2 to q3 2006.

---

[18] A few modifications have been made for Figure 4.3.1-2: for a better distinction of inputs and outputs the zero line for CI has been moved to "3". Moreover the average CCD and CCP have been divided by 100 to plot them in the same graph.

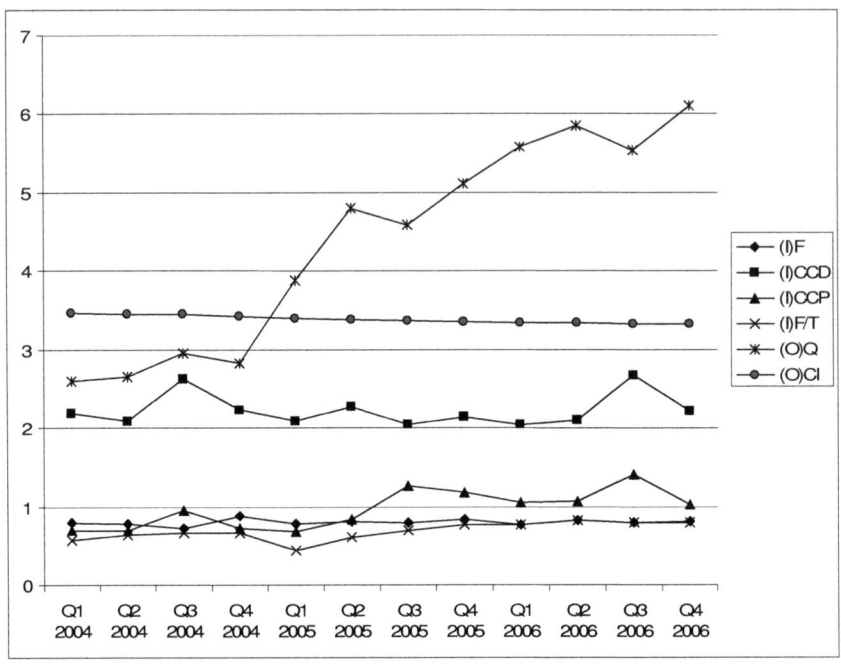

Figure 4.3.1-2: Development of average input and output values over *time (For reason of graphical illustration: CCD and CCP divided by 100; CI plus 3)*[19]

The MPI in Table 4.3.1-5 from q1 2004 to q4 2006 confirms the assumptions stated above. On average, the productivity increased from quarter to quarter by 9%.

Another inter-temporal aspect is the progress of average efficiency. Regarding the relative efficiency scores no proposition concerning the productivity development can be made because the scores are calculated separately for each quarter. Therefore, no matter how high/low the productivity of a sample is, DEA will always identify efficient and inefficient. Yet, statements like: "if the average relative efficiency in quarter x would have been higher, the productivity development of quarter x in comparison to quarter y would have been better", can be proposed.

---

[19] The corresponding data set can be found in appendix C

Malmquist	Average	Median	Max	Min	SD
q12004=>q22004	1.02	1.00	2.09	0.49	0.26
q22004=>q32004	1.01	0.95	2.02	0.47	0.30
q32004=>q42004	0.98	0.96	5.10	0.43	0.58
q42004=>q12005	1.51	1.50	2.66	0.21	0.45
q12005=>q22005	0.99	0.96	2.06	0.35	0.34
q22005=>q32005	0.84	0.84	1.79	0.17	0.25
q32005=>q42005	1.35	0.97	22.89	0.46	2.81
q42005=>q12006	1.14	1.18	2.35	0.06	0.37
q12006=>q22006	0.99	0.95	4.19	0.40	0.47
q22006=>q32006	0.92	0.88	2.83	0.24	0.34
q32006=>q42006	1.26	1.23	1.84	0.30	0.27

Table 4.3.1-5: Average productivity development described by the average MPI

Table 4.3.1-6 displays the results for the average relative efficiency development for the current DEA setting. The average relative efficiency scores vary between 64% and 78% and from the efficiency scores no statement regarding the productivity development over time can be stated. These realized efficiency scores indicate that the performance of the sales force can be improved and the efficiency score variations from one year to another can be harmonized.

Quarters	Ø Efficiency
q1 2004	67%
q2 2004	68%
q3 2004	77%
q4 2004	69%
q1 2005	78%
q2 2005	64%
q3 2005	72%
q4 2005	77%
q1 2006	76%
q2 2006	68%
q3 2006	72%
q4 2006	73%

Table 4.3.1-6: Development of Ø efficiency

The only way to improve overall relative efficiency per period and productivity from period to period is to apply a fine tuning to the individual sales reps.

This task can be achieved by an inter-temporal evaluation of each of the individuals which will be carried out in the next section.

Benchmarking of individual sales reps

Corresponding to chapter 4.1 and 4.2 sales reps 4, 28 and 42 are used to demonstrate fine tuning possibilities and the impact of changes in the DEA arrangement on an individual level for each of the SBM DEA versions. In addition to chapter 4.1 and 4.2, inter-temporal aspects, such as relative efficiency development and the MPI per individual will be assessed. Furthermore, the efficiency scores are decomposed into the different elements to evaluate the sources and magnitudes of inefficiency regarding the respective inputs and outputs for a single sales rep.
In addition, chapter 4.3 includes information about super efficiency of efficient sales reps as explained in chapter 2.4.4. This information is used to rank the efficient sales reps and for the calculation of the MPI.

The results for sales rep 4 are displayed in Figure 4.3.1-3. The efficiency score of 129% indicates SR 4 as the most efficient sales rep of the whole sample. Because SR 4 is efficient no benchmark partners are considered to evaluate SR 4. In fact SR 4 is used as benchmark partner for other inefficient units. SR 4 is mentioned 34 times as mentor in the benchmark sets of inefficient sales reps. Regarding the frequency, SR 4 is the most mentioned mentor of the 17 efficient units in benchmark sets of the inefficient sales reps. Therefore SR 4 is number one in the category frequency. Another aspect is the impact (or weights of the envelopment problem) with which SR 4 is mentioned in the benchmark sets. As mentioned in chapter 2 the magnitude of the weight determines how important a benchmark partner is for the evaluation of an inefficient sales rep.

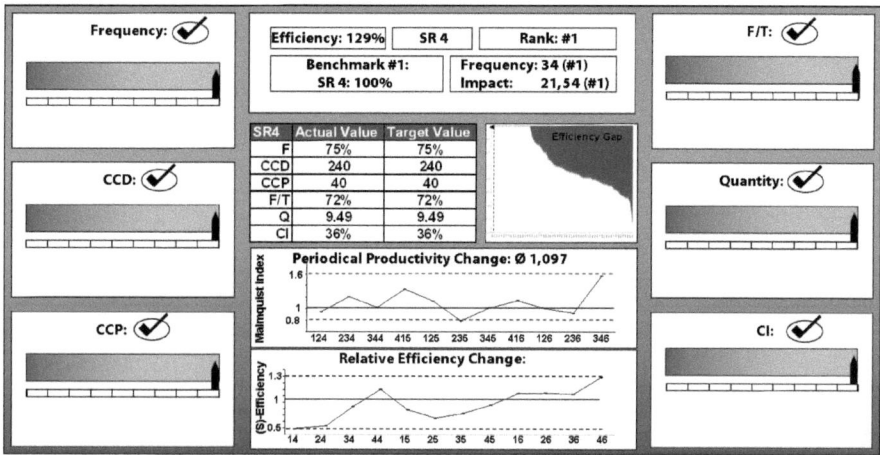

Figure 4.3.1-3: KPI-Cockpit for SR 4

Therefore cumulated weights of an efficient sales rep give information over the influence or impact of a sales rep on the sample. For SR 4 the cumulated weights account to 21.54 which places SR 4 in the top position regarding the impact on the field.

To check whether or not the results of the fourth quarter 2006 are an exception to the rule or not, the two graphs in the lower middle of Figure 4.3.1-3 can be analyzed. A first glance provides the information that the average productivity of SR 4 increased by nearly 10% per quarter. That means that the distance between input and output levels increased. This goes in line with the findings from above regarding the whole sample.

A look at the relative efficiency development over time indicates that SR 4 is following a stable upward trend since the second quarter 2005.

Putting it in a nutshell SR 4 indeed seems to be one of the best sales reps in the field not only due to the performance in the last quarter 2006 but also concerning the inter-temporal development. Henceforth, SR 4 can be recommended as mentor for inefficient sales reps. However, the present results only count for the *current DEA setting* of chapter 4.3.1.

Figure 4.3.1-4 displays the decomposition of the MPI to reveal sources of productivity growth. On the abscissa the change from quarter to quarter is depicted for the MPI (q12004=>q22004 and so on). Attributing the fact that relative efficiency is measured per period and that there are only 11 time switches the efficiency score for q1 2004 is not depicted. The first point of the efficiency on the left marks the second quarter 2004 and the last point on the right hand side marks the last quarter 2006. The catch up process (CU) (diamonds), the frontier shift (FS) (squares), the MPI (triangles) and the efficiency development (crosses) are depicted. The relation between the efficiency development and the CU is clear. As soon as the CU has a value over one, the efficiency rises, otherwise it decreases.

The MPI does not only depend on the CU but also on the frontier shift in the projection region. If the frontier from one period to another is unchanged and the CU increases, the MPI increases as well. If the frontier shift in the projection region is beneath one the MPI of a sales rep may rise or fall, depending on which effect prevails: the CU or the FS?

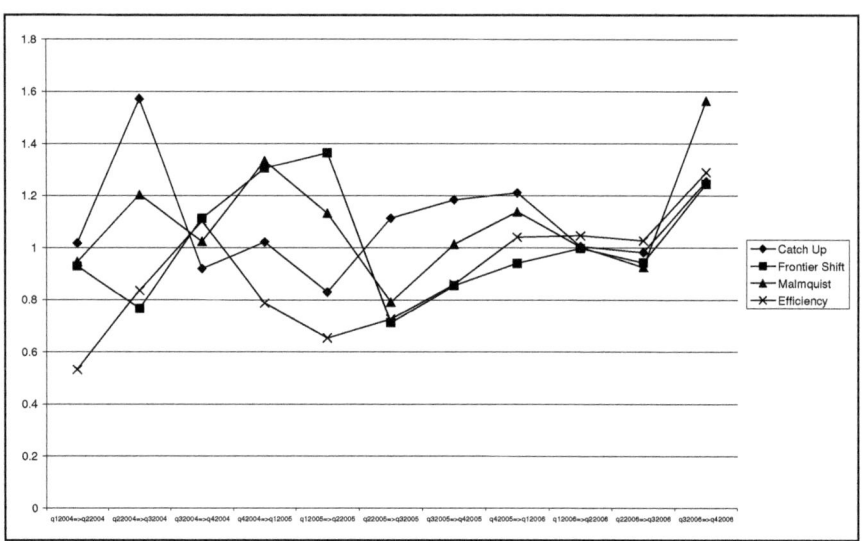

Figure 4.3.1-4: Decomposition of the MPI and presentation of the development of relative efficiency

For SR4 the efficiency development is very promising. From the beginning of the observation period the relative efficiency could be increased from about 0.54 to 1.29 in the last quarter. At the beginning of the interval the efficiency improvement is due to a high CU which indicates that SR4 is closing up to the efficiency frontier. The efficiency frontier is decreasing which indicates that the benchmark partners of SR4 in the projection region are loosing productivity. But SR4 is not influenced by that development and improves the productivity of operation from q1 2004 to q2 2004 which is indicated by an MPI>1. As SR4 reaches an efficient status, the movement CU, FS, MPI and efficiency converge because SR4 is part of the efficiency frontier.

Figure 4.3.1-5 shows the results for SR 28. With a score of 67% SR 28 is inefficient and is ranked on position #32. The most important benchmark partner of SR 28 is SR 4 with an impact of 70%. The second important is SR 32 with an impact of 30%. The input and output boxes on the right and left of Figure 4.3.1-5 indicate the percentage change in each category necessary for being efficient. On the input side for example CCP should be reduced by 45% and the Q should be increased by 41%. For SR 28 those two categories reveal the biggest percentage changes.

Furthermore the contribution of these input and output excesses to the calculated efficiency score is displayed at the bottom of each input and output box. The contribution of each input and output is calculated by the decomposition of the efficiency scores as explained in chapter two[20]. The decomposition of the efficiency score of SR 28 reveals that the biggest contribution to inefficiency is made by Q, followed by CCP. This finding concludes that the most important adjustment for SR 28 to reach efficiency is to increase the insulin sales followed by a decrease of CCP.

Concerning the average productivity increase by 5.4% of SR 28 per quarter compared to the average of 9% per quarter for the whole sample, SR 28 underperformed and has to improve. The best productivity improvement was reached from quarter 4 2004 to quarter 1 2005.
At the same time SR 28 reached 100% efficiency for one period (q1 2005). Unfortunately this top quarter was followed by a sharp decrease of efficiency and since q2 2005 the efficiency score of SR 28 moved sidewise between 60% and 80%.
This development is not really satisfying and therefore SR 28 should try to improve those parameters which were indicated to have the biggest influence on the efficiency score, namely Q and CCP.

---

[20] Decomposition for SR 28: Efficiency score of $0.67=(1-0.0163-0.0000-0.1132-0.022)/(1+0.2073+0.0559)$ → the decomposition is a weighted relation between the slack and the original data (see chapter two)

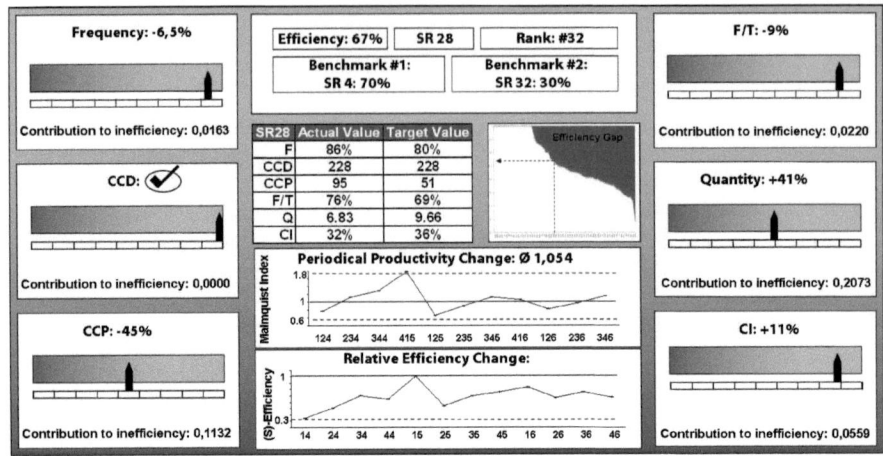

Figure 4.3.1-5: KPI-Cockpit for SR 28

Attributing the relative efficiency, SR28 is in a side movement. The efficiency score remains most of the time between 0.7 and 0.8. Due to the overall market development the MPI increases on average by 1.054. Therefore relative efficiency was unchanged but the productivity increased.

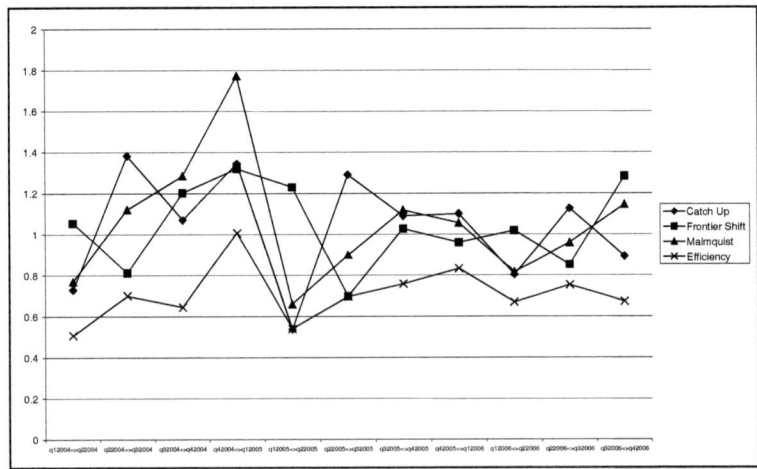

Figure 4.3.1-6: Decomposition of the MPI and presentation of the development of relative efficiency

In the first quarter 2005 (4) SR28 is efficient and the preceding periods were characterized by an impressive CU and productivity improvement. However, SR28 could not maintain this development and fell back again.

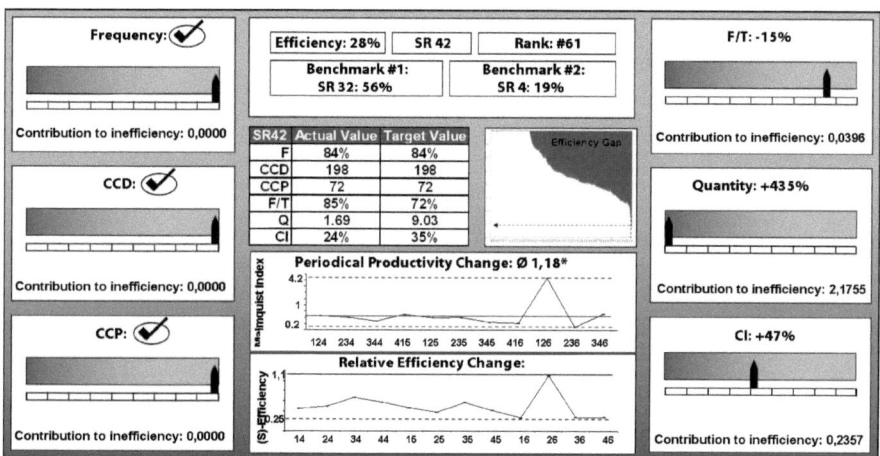

Figure 4.3.1-7: KPI-Cockpit for SR 42

As Figure 4.3.1-7 depicts SR 42 reached an efficiency score of 28% and is ranked number #61. The two most important benchmarks for SR 42 are SR 32 with 56% and SR 4 with 19%. Compared to the other sales reps the input side of SR 42 is ok, only F/T needs slight improvement. A look at the output side reveals that SR 42 needs very strong improvement. The amount insulin sold must rise by not more than 435% to reach a level that justifies the effort invested.

The decomposition of the efficiency score assigns the highest contribution to the inefficiency of SR 42 to the output Q followed by CI, as expected.

Figure 4.3.1-8 the inter-temporal analysis has to be taken into account very carefully for SR 42. The productivity development from q1 to q2 2006 is marked by a high peak with an MPI of 4.3. This is due to a job rotation. In q1 2006 another sales rep was assigned for the job of SR 42. Unfortunately the author of this thesis does not know who replaced whom and only has information over who left the overall sales force and who joined it. Therefore the job of SR 42 was reassigned by the author to a sales rep who joined the sales force in the beginning of 2006. Therefore these extreme values came up. Thus, the inter-temporal development can not be consistently tracked back to the q1 2004. However, if the sales rep replacing the job of SR 42 at the beginning of 2006 is known, the MPI and the efficiency development give valuable information whether or not the reassignment of the job was successful. Due to the job reassignment the average MPI is very high and therefore must be seen as an outlier.

The efficiency development is characterized by an extreme peak in q2 2006 as well. This happened due to the previous reasoning concerning the job rotation. In the progress of the year 2006 the efficiency score dropped to a very low level which indicates a need for very strong improvement for SR 42.

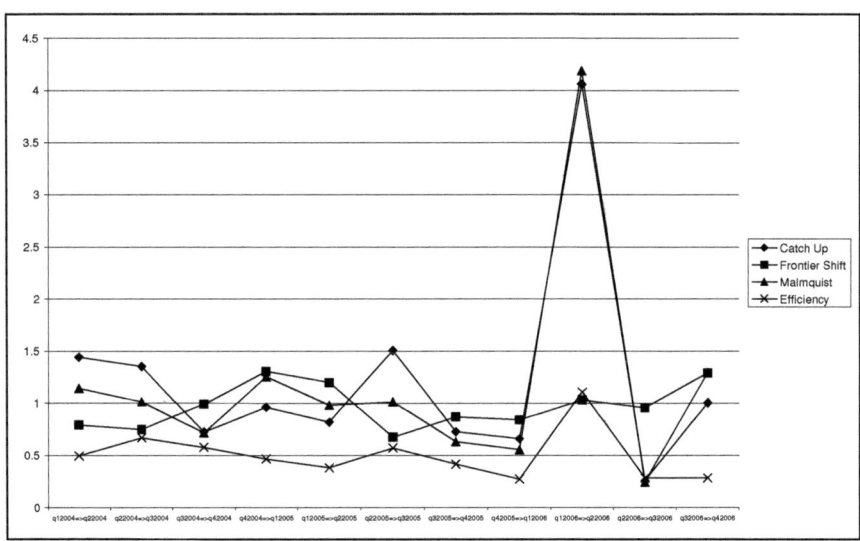

Figure 4.3.1-8: Decomposition of the MPI and presentation of the development of relative efficiency

4.3.2 SBM Model Version 2 (F, CCD, F/T, - Q, CI)

In this chapter a DEA version with F, CCD and F/T as inputs and Q and CI as outputs is presented. The efficiency gap in Figure 4.3.2-1 is presented first.

The Efficiency Gap

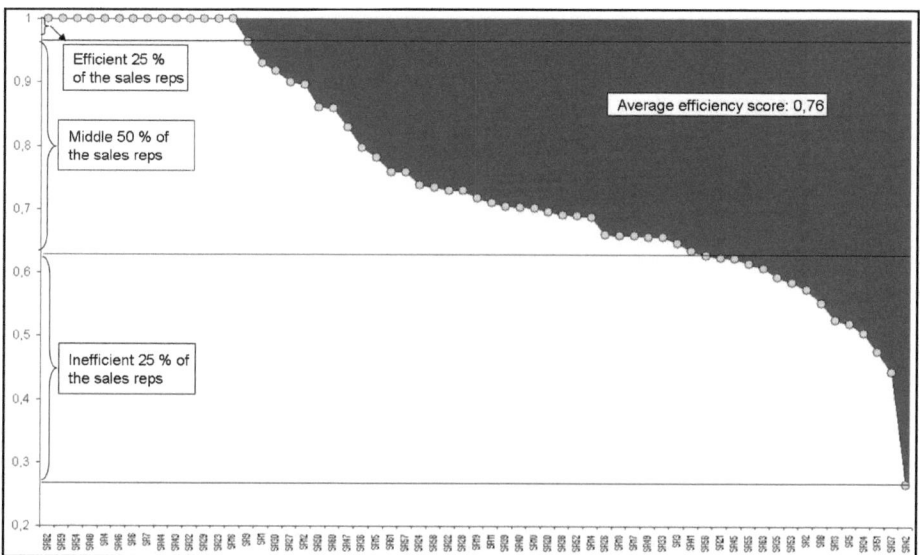

Figure 4.3.2-1: Illustration of the Efficiency Gap and of the three efficiency groups

The efficiency gap ranges from 0.27 to 1. The average efficiency score of the sample is 0.76. Due to the reduction of the DEA setting to five dimensions (CCP is excluded) the number of efficient units decreases to 14 which are less than the number of efficient units in DEA settings with six dimension (chapter 4.3.*1).

F,CCD,F/T – Q,CI Group	Average SBM-NO-V Efficiency	Average BCC-O Efficiency	Average CCR-O Efficiency
Efficient 25%	100%	100%	100%
Middle 50%	75%	88%	83%
Inefficient 25%	54%	68%	64%

Table 4.3.2-1: Comparison of average efficiency scores

Turning to Table 4.3.2-1 in the SBM model, the efficient 25% reach 100% efficiency, the middle 50% achieve an average efficiency score of 75% and the inefficient 25% reach an average score of 54%. Compared to the corresponding DEA setting calculated with the BCC and CCR model, the SBM version reveals itself to be the strictest efficiency measure, albeit the number of efficient sales reps in the SBM version of Table 4.3.2-1 is higher (14) than in the corresponding CCR version (9).

The results of the group characteristics regarding the specific input and output dimensions are displayed in Table 4.3.2-2.

- ➢ In the present DEA setting with three inputs and two outputs no significant difference on a level $p \leq 5\%$ concerning the input frequency is detected. The only statement possible is to conclude that the efficient 25% use the input frequency more efficiently than the middle group for a level of significance of $p \leq 10\%$.

- ➢ The input CCD shows no statistical significant difference between the groups. Hence, on a global level, CCD has a similar effect on efficiency in all quartiles.

- ➢ The input F/T is characterized by significant differences between the efficient group and the other two groups. The efficient group has a mean rank for a F/T unit that is higher than in the other two groups. This outcome points out that the efficient group generates more output from their portion of fixed doctor relations compared to the other groups. The difference between the middle and the low group is not significant.

- ➢ The output Q of the top group reaches a significantly higher mean rank per unit than the other groups. This fact concludes that the efficient 25% produce more Q from less input than the other two groups do. The middle and the inefficient group have similar virtual prices and, therefore, the mean ranks do not differ significantly. Henceforth, no distinction concerning the output Q between the middle 50% and the inefficient 25% can be made.

Input/Output	Group	Group Average Weights	Mean Rank	z-value	doublesided p-value
Frequency	efficient 25%	1.06	28.3	1.66	0.0969
	middle 50%	0.4	21.2		
	efficient 25%	1.3	17.4	1.14	0.2543
	inefficient 25%	0.54	13.6		
	middle 50%	0.4	22.5	-0.71	0.4777
	inefficient 25%	0.54	25.6		
CCD	efficient 25%	0.00402	25.8	0.8	0.4237
	middle 50%	0.00281	22.4		
	efficient 25%	0.00402	17.3	1.08	0.2801
	inefficient 25%	0.00195	13.7		
	middle 50%	0.00281	24.5	0.71	0.4777
	inefficient 25%	0.00195	21.4		
F/T	efficient 25%	2.29432	29.6	2.13	0.0332
	middle 50%	0,62349	20.5		
	efficient 25%	2.29432	20.3	2.97	0.003
	inefficient 25%	0.40379	10.7		
	middle 50%	0.62349	24.4	0.61	0.5419
	inefficient 25%	0.40379	21.7		
Q	efficient 25%	0.13	35.5	4.22	<.0001
	middle 50%	0.06	17.7		
	efficient 25%	0.13	21.7	3.82	0.0001
	inefficient 25%	0.06	9.3		
	middle 50%	0.06	23.00	-0.35	0.7263
	inefficient 25%	0.06	24.5		
CI	efficient 25%	5.88	33.4	3.47	0.0005
	middle 50%	2.73	18.7		
	efficient 25%	5.88	21.9	3.94	0.0001
	inefficient 25%	1.26	9.1		
	middle 50%	2.73	26.9	2.46	0.0139
	inefficient 25%	1.26	16.5		

Table 4.3.2-2: Relationship between average efficiency scores and input and output multipliers

➢ The competition index reveals clear differences between all of the groups. The efficient 25% face competition in the best way, followed by the middle group and then the inefficient group. The top group has the highest virtual prices followed by the middle group. The inefficient 25% are assigned the lowest virtual price.

A summary of the points mentioned above gives rise to the conclusion that higher Q, higher CI and lower F/T are the keys for increasing efficiency *in this setting*. CCD and F for instance seem to have a minor effect on efficiency.

Groups	F	CCD	F/T	Q	CI
efficient 25%	0.73	0.68	1.28	0.87	1.93
middle 50%	0.44	0.62	0.48	0.37	0.77
inefficient 25%	0.45	0.41	0.33	0.27	0.38

Table 4.3.2-3: Average virtual worth of the input or output category

The results of Table 4.3.2-3 shed light on the question where to adjust inputs and outputs first. Due to the fact that the results of the middle group are not so straight forward because the differences of the virtual worth between the dimensions are not so distinctive and considering the fact that the optimization potential is not as big as in the inefficient group, the author concentrates on the conclusion stemming from the inefficient group.

Regarding the fact that a low virtual worth in comparison to the virtual worth of the other dimensions of a group indicates great efficiency potential, the inefficient group would be well advised to increase the quantity insulin sold on the output side first and decreasing and improving the quality of F/T and CCD on the input side secondly.

This conclusion is supported by the results of Table 4.3.2-4. The table displays the overall reductions of CCD of 7.7%, the reduction of F/T of 14% and the increase of Q to 37%. The optimal frequency is calculated to be 80%, which is the same target as set for sales reps by the company[21]. The optimal F/T is 69%, which is 11% lower than the company internal target.

Input/Output	Actual Value	Target Value	Delta %
Ø F	81%	80%	-1%
CCD	13517	12471	-7.7%
Ø F/T	80%	69%	-14%
Q	373	511	37%
SOM	31%	41%	10%

Table 4.3.2-4: Comparison of current and optimal target values

The amount of insulin sold should be increased by 138 MMU per quarter to reach an efficient level. This increase of MMU sales would correspond to a market share increase of 10%.

Examining a single time period is fine for an analysis of the status quo. But perhaps it is of additional worth to check long term developments in order to make strategic conclusions.

---

[21] The target for every sales rep set up for the company internal benchmark is 80%.

Inter-temporal Aspects

Figure 4.3.2-2 tracks the input and output development for this DEA setting. The input CCP is not displayed.

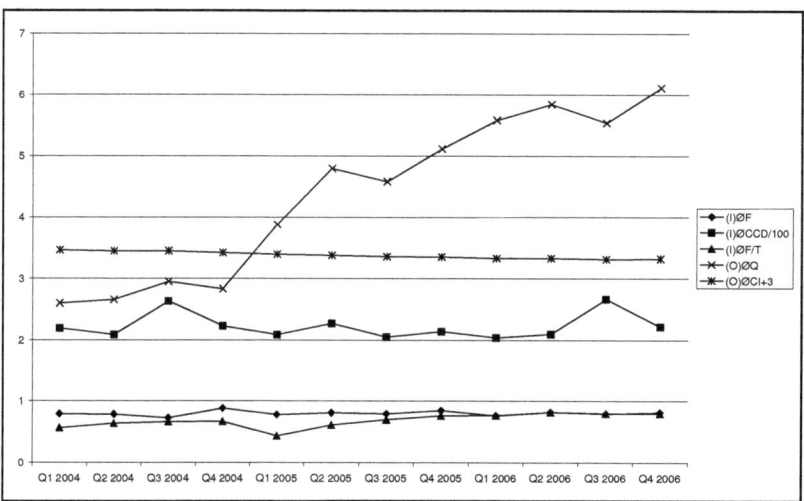

Figure 4.3.2-2: Development of average input and output values over *time (For reason of graphical illustration: CCD divided by 100; CI plus 3)*

For this setting, with CCP missing, a long term productivity increase can be observed, as already noticed in the previous chapter. A first analysis leads to the assumption that the MPI decreased at least from q3 to q4 2004, from q2 to q3 2004 and from q2 to q3 2006 because both outputs decreased and the inputs did not fall significantly.

This assumption is supported by Table 4.3.2-5. In addition to the time periods mentioned above, the MPI falls from q3 to q4 2005 and from q1 to q2 2006. A closer look at Figure 4.3.2-2 reveals that the average amount of inputs increased in the mentioned periods which probably outbalanced the insulin sales growth and, therefore, resulted in a MPI<1.

Malmquist	Average	Median	Max	Min	SD
q12004=>q22004	1,01	1,00	2,01	0,50	0,25
q22004=>q32004	1,09	1,03	2,18	0,66	0,28
q32004=>q42004	0,88	0,88	2,53	0,40	0,28
q42004=>q12005	1,49	1,46	2,74	0,45	0,43
q12005=>q22005	1,02	0,97	2,32	0,35	0,35
q22005=>q32005	0,96	0,96	1,65	0,16	0,22
q32005=>q42005	0,97	0,95	1,67	0,48	0,23
q42005=>q12006	1,14	1,13	2,02	0,52	0,28
q12006=>q22006	0,99	0,95	4,16	0,39	0,44
q22006=>q32006	0,96	0,92	2,68	0,23	0,32
q32006=>q42006	1,16	1,12	1,66	0,32	0,22

Table 4.3.2-5: Average productivity development described by the overall MPI

The median values follow the same trend as the average values and confirms the productivity development. There are some extreme values like a max MPI of 4.16 accompanied by a higher standard deviation. In this case the outlier is SR 42. The reason for the outbreak has been explained further above.

The efficiency development in Table 4.3.2-6 shows that the average efficiency score varied between 0.62 and 0.77. This finding is similar to the previous chapter and gives the information that there still is a great potential for improvement within the sales force.

Quarters	Ø Efficiency
q1 2004	0,67
q2 2004	0,66
q3 2004	0,77
q4 2004	0,69
q1 2005	0,76
q2 2005	0,62
q3 2005	0,72
q4 2005	0,73
q1 2006	0,76
q2 2006	0,68
q3 2006	0,72
q4 2006	0,76

Table 4.3.2-6: Development of Ø efficiency

Of course this improvement of the overall sales force has to be achieved on an individual level as presented in the next section for the current DEA setting.

Benchmarking of individual sales reps

Using SR 4, 28 and 42 as examples the impact of reduction of the dimensions to three inputs will be analysed. Figure 4.3.2-3 displays the KPI-Cockpit for SR 4 with an efficiency score of 104%. In this setting SR 4 is not the best anymore and is ranked as #4. Furthermore, the importance of SR4 as benchmark for inefficient sales reps decreased in comparison to the case where CCP was included as input. SR 4 is only used as benchmark for one other sales rep and for itself. Therefore, the impact on the sample is very low and SR 4 takes the thirteenth place within the group of efficient sales reps.

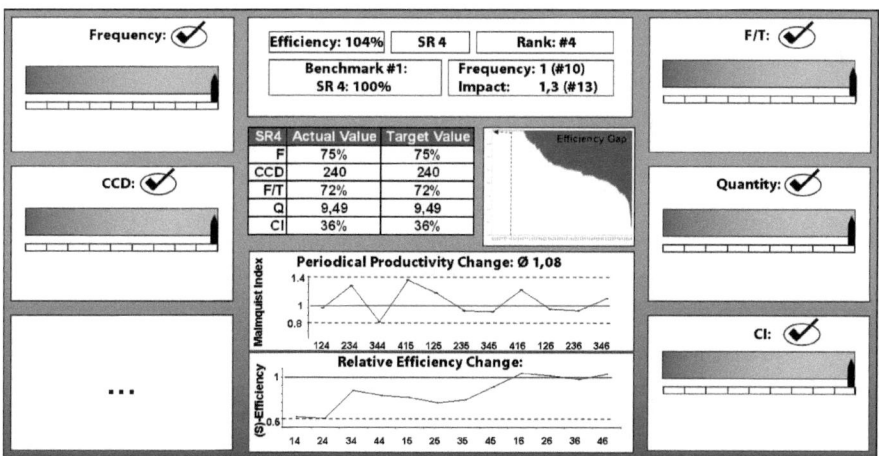

Figure 4.3.2-3: KPI-Cockpit for SR 4 (F, CCD, F/T – Q,CI)

Because SR4 is efficient all the input and output categories are fine. The MPI of SR4 increased by about 8% per quarter. The development of relative efficiency is very good and SR4 has been working efficient since the beginning of 2006. To conclude the reduction of the dimensions by CCP reduced SR4 overall performance. Hence, CCP contributed positively to SR 4 efficiency calculation which in turn means that SR 4s use of CCP was exemplary.

A more detailed analysis of the inter-temporal development is presented in Figure 4.3.2-4.

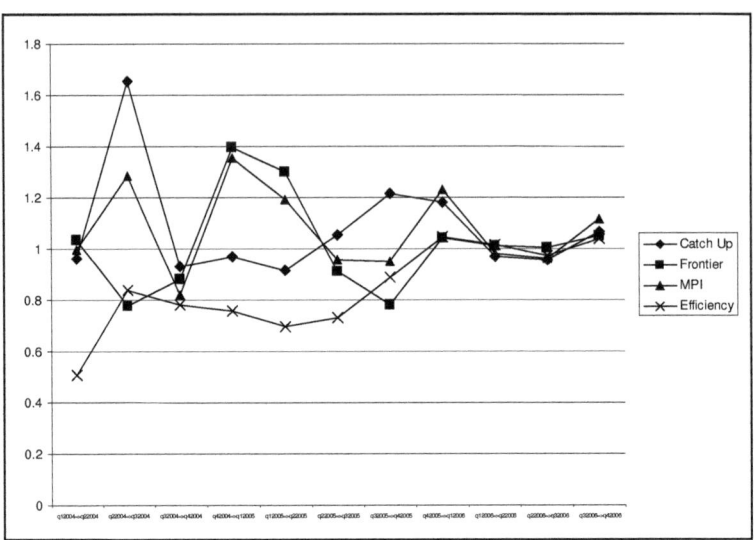

Figure 4.3.2-4: Decomposition of the MPI and the efficiency development of SR4

From q2 2004 to q3 2004 efficiency increased and SR4 approached the efficiency frontier fast. Therefore the CU is fairly high. Unfortunately, the frontier technology around SR4 retreated and, therefore, has a negative effect on SR4s MPI. Henceforth, the productivity increase of SR4 was negatively influenced by the frontier drawback and positively influenced by the increasing efficiency of SR4.

In this setting SR4 undergoes an almost ideal development. Starting off with a low efficiency score in q2 2004 (q1 2004 is not displayed) SR4 is moving closer and closer towards the efficiency frontier. At the beginning, the CU is fairly high and is converging against zero in the end. The same counts for the MPI which oscillates around one and converges against one with an average score above one. The frontier shifts similarly and is slightly above one which indicates that the efficient sales reps in the projection region increase their productivity from period to period.

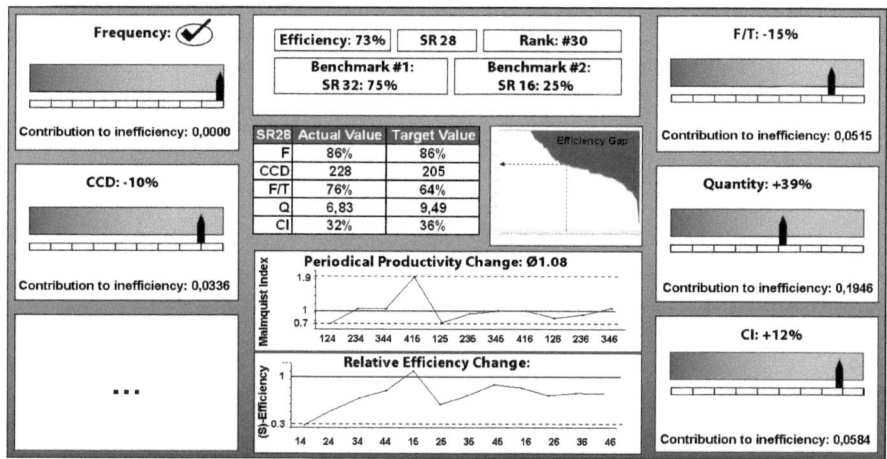

Figure 4.3.2-5: KPI-Cockpit for SR 28 (F, CCD, F/T – Q,CI)

The situation for SR28 is very different. SR4 is exposed to a negative effect on efficiency through the exclusion of CCP, but SR28 experienced a positive effect on the efficiency score which increases to 73%. In addition SR28 moves up two places to rank #30. The main benchmark partners for SR28 are SR32 with 75% and SR16 with 25%. The input F is fine. The other two inputs need slight improvement. The main source of inefficiency is on the output side. This can be concluded after summing up the contribution of the input side to inefficiency (0.0851) and the contribution of the output side to inefficiency (0.2530). Therefore, the most potential for improvement regarding efficiency is detected on the output side. Especially the output Q has to be improved by 39% from 6.83 MMU to 9.49 MMU sold to reach an efficient level.

In this DEA version SR28 reaches a stable efficiency score between 70% and 80% over the period of time with an average MPI of 1.08. Therefore, SR28 is becoming more productive but on the same relative efficiency level. Thus, SR28 should try to increase efficiency, which in turn would improve productivity. In fact, this means that SR28 more or less has the same distance to the frontier as the frontier shifts outwards (efficient SRs are getting more productive) during the periods. This expresses itself by a CU closely around one and an MPI moving close too the FS.

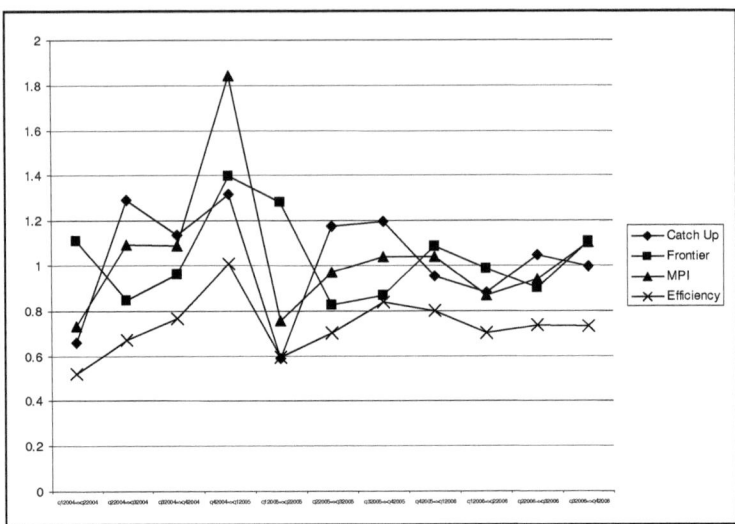
Figure 4.3.2-6: Decomposition of the MPI and the efficiency development of SR28

Figure 4.3.2-6 supports this assumption. In the last four quarters the CUP is shifting around one and the MPI is moving close to the FS. Therefore the efficiency score remains on a level between 70% and 80%. The most effective way for SR28 to reach the efficiency frontier for SR28 is to start to increase the amount MMU sold because this output dimension is responsible for the most of the inefficiency of SR28 as Figure 4.3.2-5 shows.

For SR42 the present DEA version calculated a slightly lower efficiency score of 27% in comparison to the version including CCP as depicted in Figure 4.3.2-7. Therefore, SR42 retains the last position and is ranked #61. The most important benchmark is SR 32 with 80% and SR2 with 20%. The two inputs F and CCD are fine but the input F/T could be improved. The result of this finding is that SR42 should use less fixed doctor relations in order to produce more output. Hence the quality of these long term doctor relations should be improved or, on the other hand, the social skills of SR42.

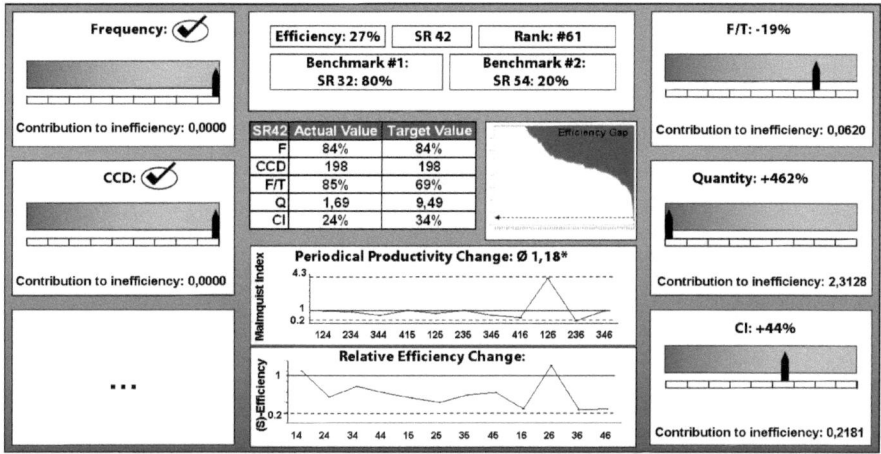

Figure 4.3.2-7: KPI-Cockpit for SR 28 (F, CCD, F/T – Q, CI)

On the output side the amount of insulin sold (Q) should be increased to 9.49 and the CI should rise to 34%. These two numbers indicate that SR42 is on a very low output level compared to the effort invested. The contribution to inefficiency from the input side amounts to 0.062 and from the output side 2.5309. Therefore, the major source of inefficiency is on the output side for SR42.

The inter-temporal development for SR42 does not look very promising. Except for a peak in the second quarter 2006 (which is an outlier, see discussion above) the efficiency development is decreasing steadily. Because of the mentioned outlier the average MPI is calculated to be 1.18. If the MPI of SR42 is adjusted[22] for the outlier, the average MPI is beneath one which gives the information of a decreasing productivity from quarter to quarter. Therefore a final conclusion on the future of SR42 cannot be better than in the version 1 with CCP as additional input. SR42 needs to improve greatly or perhaps should leave the company.

---

[22] This adjustment is exemplary and is only undertaken in this subchapter for clarification reasons.

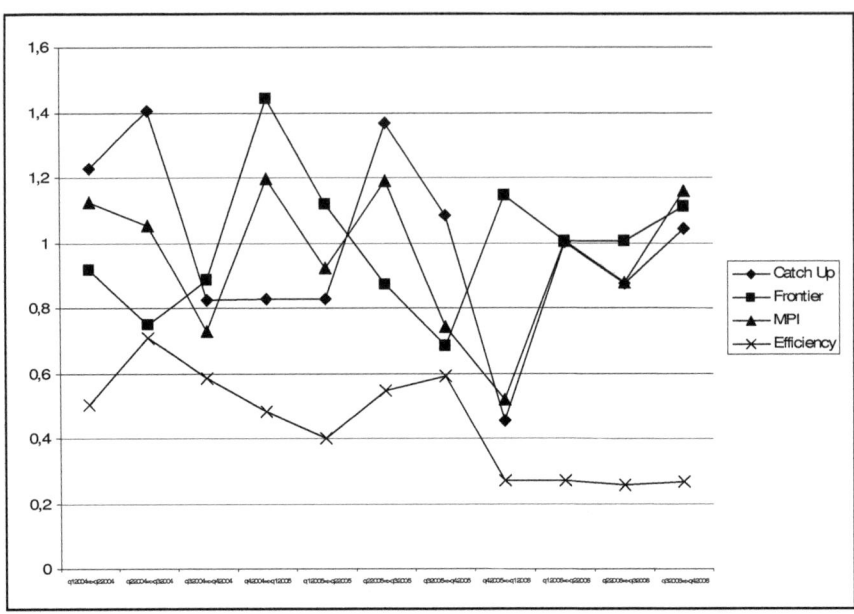

Figure 4.3.2-8: Decomposition of the MPI and the efficiency development of SR42 *(adjusted for the outlier in q12006→q22006)*

The decomposition of the MPI in Figure 4.3.2-8 gives the details. The CU is mainly smaller than one which resolves in the downward trend of efficiency. For the frontier in the projection region no clear trend can be detected. The average frontier shift is slightly under one and therefore is more or less stable over time. The average MPI adjusted for the outlier from q1 2006 to q2 2006 (MPI, CU and FS were set to one→ no change) calculates to 0.89 which indicates a sharp decrease in productivity.

4.3.3 SBM Model Version 3 (F, CCD, CCP, F/T - SOM)

In this DEA version only the market share is viewed as output and the input side is determined by the four inputs F, CCD, CCP and F/T.

The Efficiency Gap

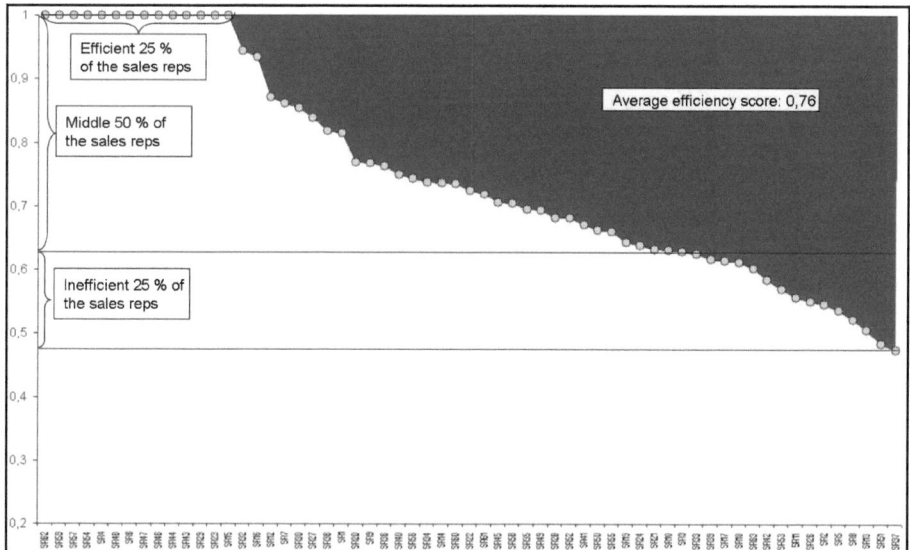

Figure 4.3.3-1: Illustration of the Efficiency Gap and of the three efficiency groups

In this DEA setting the spread of the efficiency gap is smaller than in the chapters 4.3.1 – 2 and ranges between 0.48 and 1. The average efficiency score calculates to 0.76 where 15 sales reps reach an efficient status. Table 4.3.3-1 depicts the average efficiency scores attained by the three different groups for the three different DEA models. The SBM model is the strictest efficiency measure regarding the middle and inefficient group.

F,CCD,CCP, F/T – SOM Group	Average SBM-NO-V Efficiency	Average BCC-O Efficiency	Average CCR-O Efficiency
Efficient 25%	100%	100%	97%
Middle 50%	73%	84%	79%
Inefficient 25%	56%	65%	61%

Table 4.3.3-1: Comparison of average efficiency scores

Due to the assumption of CRS in the CCR model, the amount of efficient units in that model reaches 8. Therefore, units with an efficiency score less than 1 belong to the top 25% and, therefore, the average score is lower than 100%.

Table 4.3.3-2 tries to identify the reasons for a high efficiency score regarding the output and input categories.

- In this DEA setting no significant characteristics regarding the weights of input F can be distinguished.

- The input CCD reveals that virtual weights (prices) for this category differ significantly between the top and the middle group with $p \leq 10\%$, and between the top and the inefficient group with $p \leq 5\%$. This finding shows that the top group uses CCD more intensely than the others and therefore the marginal return of one call to doctors considering the market share is higher. Between the middle and the low group no significant distinction is found.

- A similar conclusion holds for the input CCP. Again the top group has higher virtual price of CCP than the other two groups and, therefore, it uses the best portion of CCP in relation to the output compared to the other two groups. Between the middle and the low group no significant distinction is found.

- The amount of fixed doctor relation has a significantly different effect on efficiency between the groups. The top group uses the existing long term doctor relations very efficiently in the sense that they can profit the most from such a relation regarding sales. This is indicated by the highest average virtual weight which is assigned to the top group. The two lower groups do not differ significantly in the category F/T.

- The most distinctive differences occur on the output side. The extremely low p-values between the top group and the two other groups lead to the statement that the market share is an important driver of efficiency.

Input/Output	Group	Group Average Weights	Mean Rank	z-value	doublesided p-value
Frequency	efficient 25%	0.44	25	0.53	0.5961
	middle 50%	0.38	22.8		
	efficient 25%	0.44	16.8	0.77	0.4413
	inefficient 25%	0.30	14.2		
	middle 50%	0.38	23.9	0.29	0.7718
	inefficient 25%	0.30	22.6		
CCD	efficient 25%	0.00507	28.5	1.73	0.0836
	middle 50%	0.00227	21.1		
	efficient 25%	0.00507	18.8	2.05	0.0404
	inefficient 25%	0.00184	12.2		
	middle 50%	0.00227	25.1	1.12	0.2627
	inefficient 25%	0.00184	20.3		
CCP	efficient 25%	0.00467	32.3	3.09	0.002
	middle 50%	0.00253	19.2		
	efficient 25%	0.00467	20	2.76	0.0058
	inefficient 25%	0.00259	11		
	middle 50%	0.00253	24.1	0.46	0.6455
	inefficient 25%	0.00259	22.2		
F/T	efficient 25%	1.84	30.8	2.57	0.0102
	middle 50%	0.47	20		
	efficient 25%	1.84	20	2.78	0.0054
	inefficient 25%	0.34	11		
	middle 50%	0.47	24.6	0.8	0.4237
	inefficient 25%	0.34	21.2		
SOM	efficient 25%	6.97	37.3	4.83	<.0001
	middle 50%	3.19	16.8		
	efficient 25%	6.97	23	4.65	<.0001
	inefficient 25%	2.07	8		
	middle 50%	3.19	25.5	1.48	0.1389
	inefficient 25%	2.07	19.3		

Table 4.3.3-2: Sources of efficiency for the different groups

Summarizing the results above, one can conclude that the input frequency is not so important for the achievement of a high efficiency score. The output SOM seems to be very important for efficiency, whereas the other three dimensions all have a similar, weaker effect on efficiency than the output SOM has. The rule is that the virtual price of an input and output unit rises as soon as these input/output units are used/produced more efficiently.

Groups	F	CCD	CCP	F/T	SOM
efficient 25%	0.30	0.88	0.40	1.11	2.61
middle 50%	0.29	0.49	0.26	0.38	0.86
inefficient 25%	0.25	0.40	0.26	0.28	0.56

Table 4.3.3-3: Average virtual worth of the input or output category

Table 4.3.3-3 presents the average virtual price times the average input and output amount in each of the categories. For the middle and inefficient groups the table shows that especially the inputs CCP and F have a very low virtual worth in comparison to the other categories. In the inefficient group the input F/T has a similar value as the categories F and CCP but in the middle group F/T clearly has a higher value than F and CCP. Therefore the greatest optimization potential on the input side is within the two categories CCP and F. On the output side only SOM can be optimized and the greatest optimization potential considering SOM is detected in the inefficient group due to the low virtual worth of this category.

The conclusion from Table 4.3.3-3 is underlined by Table 4.3.3-4, which displays the overall optimization potential. The biggest optimizations on the input side are indicated with -22% for the input CCP and -18% points for the input F. The average market share reaches an optimal level for the fourth quarter 2006 at 38%.

Input/Output	Actual Value	Target Value	Delta %
Ø F	81%	63%	-18%
CCD	13517	12975	-4%
CCP	6245	4874	-22%
Ø F/T	80%	72%	-8%
Ø SOM	31%	38%	6%

Table 4.3.3-4: Comparison of current and optimal target values

Following the analysis of the single fourth quarter 2006 the inter-temporal analysis is presented.

Inter-temporal Aspects

Figure 4.3.3-2 shows the development of the input and output categories from q1 2004 to q4 2006. The zero line for SOM has been shifted to three for reasons of better illustration. The input CCD and CCP are divided by 100.

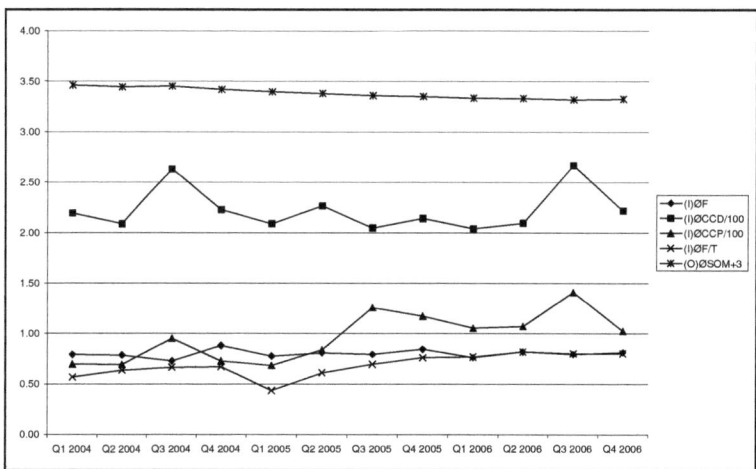

Figure 4.3.3-2: Development of average input and output values over *time (For reason of graphical illustration: CCD and CCP divided by 100 SOM plus 3)*

In contrast to the other DEA versions with the two outputs Q and CI a downward trend on the output side is detected. Due to the relatively stable input side, except for CCP which is increasing slightly, the overall productivity of the sales force should be decreasing.

This finding is supported by Table 4.3.3-5. The average MPI for the time periods displayed amounts to 0.99. Thus, the sales forces productivity decreased slightly because the relation between efforts invested and achieved SOM decreased. The median has the same tendency. The standard deviation is the highest in the third row. This is due to an outlier in the data.

Malmquist	Average	Median	Max	Min	SD
q12004=>q22004	1.00	0.98	2.55	0.57	0.32
q22004=>q32004	0.94	0.90	1.67	0.51	0.22
q32004=>q42004	0.93	0.88	5.10	0.40	0.59
q42004=>q12005	1.27	1.22	2.40	0.13	0.42
q12005=>q22005	0.82	0.79	1.62	0.43	0.22
q22005=>q32005	0.86	0.86	1.47	0.17	0.19
q32005=>q42005	0.92	0.91	1.24	0.58	0.15
q42005=>q12006	1.10	1.09	1.66	0.64	0.23
q12006=>q22006	0.94	0.90	2.29	0.45	0.28
q22006=>q32006	0.94	0.88	2.50	0.39	0.30
q32006=>q42006	1.18	1.14	1.77	0.34	0.23

Table 4.3.3-5: Average productivity development described by the overall MPI

The efficiency development of the sales force is displayed below in Table 4.3.3-6 and indicates that the sales force has still great improvement potential. The maximum average score achieved is 0.77 in q4 2005 and the lowest 0.52 in q1 2004. As stated in the other versions, the average efficiency scores still leave room for upward improvements for the sales force. For more sales success, the management has to establish an upward trend with a lower variance of the efficiency scores.

Quarters	Ø Efficiency
q1 2004	0.52
q2 2004	0.61
q3 2004	0.74
q4 2004	0.57
q1 2005	0.75
q2 2005	0.60
q3 2005	0.73
q4 2005	0.77
q1 2006	0.73
q2 2006	0.65
q3 2006	0.68
q4 2006	0.76

Table 4.3.3-6: Development of Ø efficiency

Due to the fact that the conclusions and effects on the individual level differ from the other DEA versions, the individual optimization possibilities will be regarded next.

Benchmarking of individual sales reps

Figure 4.3.2-3 displays the results for the first individual. In this setting SR4 is ranked number one again and achieves an efficiency score of 118%. Interestingly SR4 is not mentioned very often as benchmark partner for other sales rep and in addition has a low impact factor. The MPI of SR4 accounts to 0.99 and therefore the productivity of SR4 declined slightly from quarter to quarter. In the case of this sales rep efficiency over time increased despite a decreasing MPI. Hence, the benchmark partners of SR4 lost productivity faster than SR4 did. The efficiency development reveals a nice upward trend and so SR4 managed to reach an efficient status in the fourth quarter of 2006.

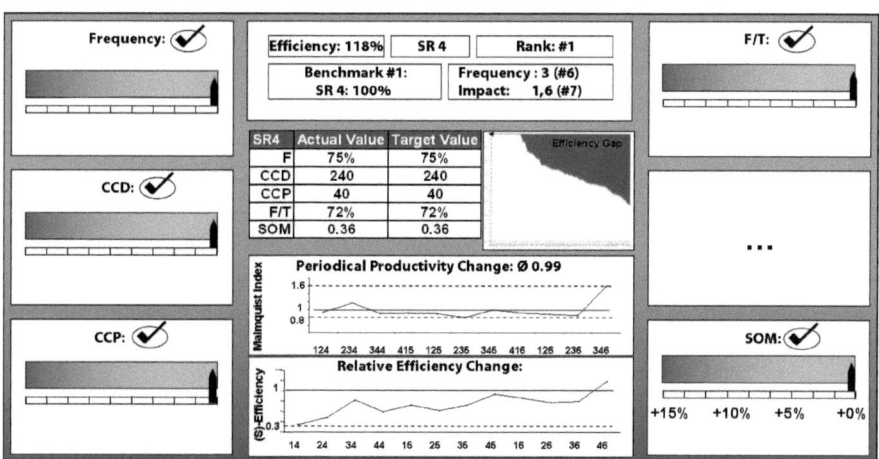

Figure 4.3.3-3: KPI-Cockpit for SR 4 (F, CCD, CCP, F/T – SOM)

In comparison to the version with F, CCD, CCP, F/T as inputs and Q and CI as outputs, sales rep 4 is still very efficient but is not mentioned as a benchmark partner frequently. This leads to the conclusion that the importance as a benchmark partner of SR4 stems from the inclusion of the absolute amount of insulin sold into the analysis. This information shows that the transformation system of inputs to outputs of SR4 is more of an exception to the rule *in this DEA setting*. The column for Q reveals that SR4 has sold the second biggest amount of insulin and, therefore, is a good example for the other sales reps in the setting with Q as output.

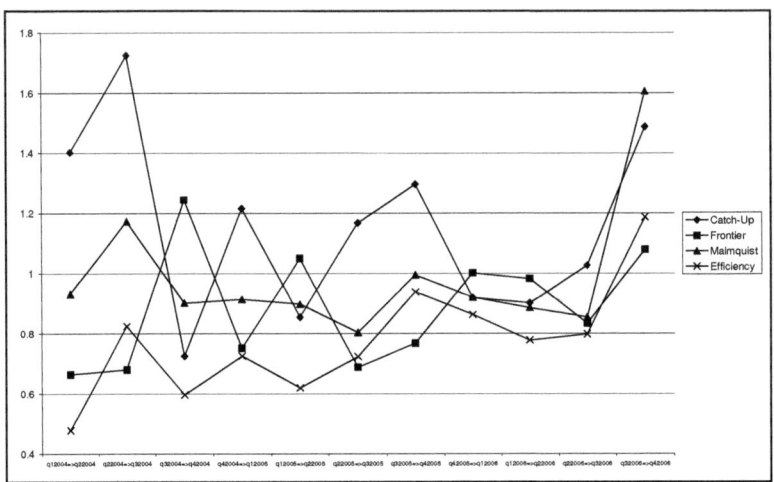

Figure 4.3.3-4: Decomposition of the MPI and the efficiency development of SR4

The decomposition of the MPI is displayed in Figure 4.3.3-4. The frontier shift (average 0.98) and the MPI are mostly beneath one which reflects on average MPI of 0.99. The CU is above one most of the time with an average value of 1.09. Hence, the efficiency of SR4 increased but total factor productivity decreased.

In Figure 4.3.3-5 SR28 reaches the rank of #37 and the efficiency score calculates to 0.68. Only SR6 is a benchmark partner for SR28. The inputs F (-41%), CCP (-20%) and F/T (-8%) need improvement as well as the output SOM (+7%points). The inefficient dimensions have contributed differently to the overall inefficiency score. On the input side, F has the highest contribution to inefficiency with 0.1017. The overall input contribution to inefficiency is 0.1714 compared to the output contribution of 0.2145. Thus, the best way for SR28 to improve the efficiency score is by an improvement of the output side. Despite an overall decreasing productivity index of the sales force, the MPI of SR28 on average, increased during the time periods of interest and, hence efficiency must have risen. The efficiency score follows an upward trend and therefore SR28 should concentrate on continuing on this promising path towards efficiency.

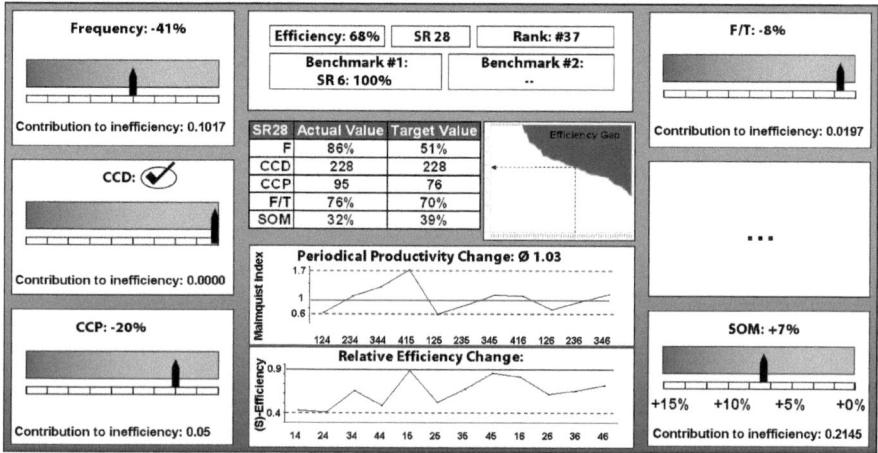

Figure 4.3.3-5: KPI-Cockpit for SR 28 (F, CCD, CCP, F/T – SOM)

Figure 4.3.3-6 depicts that the variances of the CU, the frontier shift and the MPI decrease. Due to the upward-trend of the efficiency score in this DEA setting from 0.4 to nearly 0.7, the average CU is greater than one. Therefore, SR28 is improving the sales process in comparison to its benchmark partners whom are loosing productivity, which is indicated by an average FS below one.

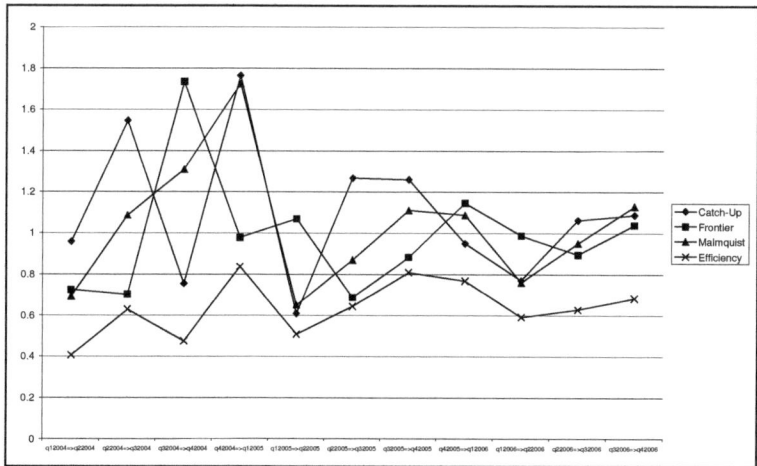

Figure 4.3.3-6: Decomposition of the MPI and the efficiency development of SR28

Last but not least, SR 42 shall be analysed for the impact of a DEA setting with SOM as output on efficiency aspects. Obviously SR42 has improved efficiency due to the rearrangement of the DEA setting and moved up to #52. The efficiency score calculates to 58%, which is much better than in the previous calculations and the main benchmark partners are SR44 (61%) and SR6 (33%).

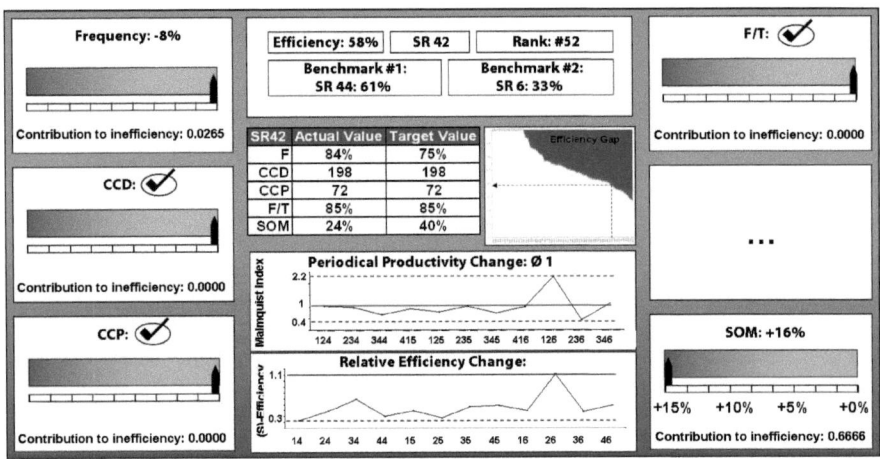

Figure 4.3.3-7: KPI-Cockpit for SR 42 (F, CCD, CCP, F/T – SOM)

The input side is fine but the market share has to be increase by 16% points to reach an efficient status. This shows that the quantities of inputs SR42 uses are fine but the quality of these inputs must be improved. The average MPI is equal to one which points out that SR42 did not improve with respect to productivity during the last twelve quarters. The average efficiency score moves between 0.5 and 0.6 except for the one outlier in q2 2006.

The decomposition of the MPI underlines the low performance of SR42. CU and FS often undergo the opposite development which results in an average MPI of one. Due to the huge improvement potential SR42 has, the efficiency score should have increased over time which would have in turn improved the MPI. Unfortunately this did not happen and therefore the status of SR42 within the company should be reconceived.

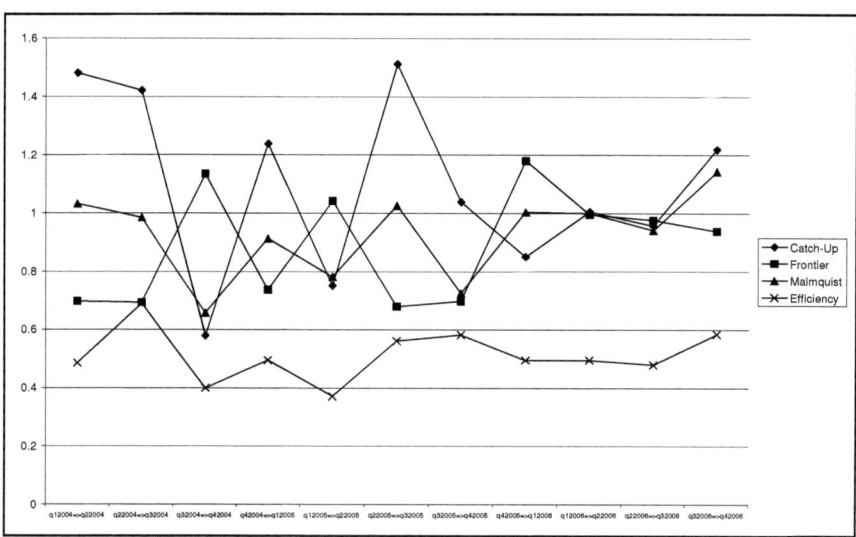

Figure 4.3.3-8: Decomposition of the MPI and the efficiency development of SR42 *(adjusted for the outlier in q12006→q22006*

4.3.4 SBM Model Version 4 (F, CCD, CCP, F/T - TR)

The following DEA version accounts for TR as a single output and F, CCD, CCP and F/T as inputs.

The Efficiency Gap

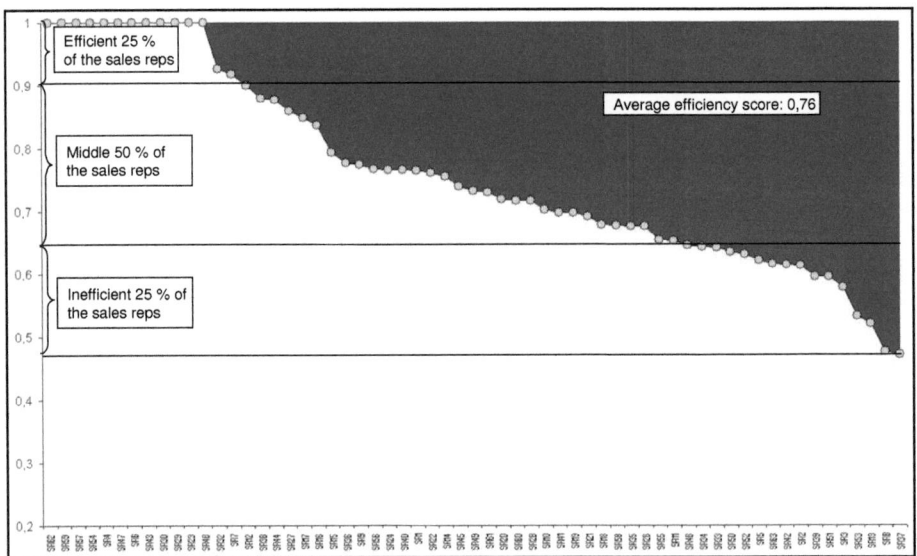

Figure 4.3.4-1: Illustration of the Efficiency Gap and of the three efficiency groups

In this DEA setting, the efficiency gap is smaller and ranges between 0.48 and 1. The average efficiency score calculates to 0.76 where 11 sales reps reach an efficient status.

Table 4.3.2-1 displays the average efficiency scores for each of the groups in the different DEA models. The average SBM efficiency scores again are the strictest ones. In none of the DEA models the top group reached an average of 100%. The average efficiency scores of the inefficient 25% are higher in each model in Table 4.3.2-1 than in the cases when Q and CI are included into the analysis. This fact shows that the output TR seems to weaken the top group and to strengthen the inefficient 25% regarding the average efficiency scores attained.

F,CCD,CCP, F/T – TR Group	Average SBM-NO-V Efficiency	Average BCC-O Efficiency	Average CCR-O Efficiency
Efficient 25%	98%	99%	98%
Middle 50%	74%	84%	79%
Inefficient 25%	64%	67%	64%

Table 4.3.4-1: Comparison of average efficiency scores

Table 4.3.4-2 seeks to identify the reasons for a high efficiency score regarding the output and input categories.

➢ As in previous DEA settings in this setting no significant characteristics regarding the weights of input F can be distinguished. This finding once again points out that there is no significant difference between the groups regarding the intensity of the use of F as a production factor.

➢ The input category CCD shows highly significant ($p \leq 5\%$) differences between the efficient 25% and the middle and inefficient group. The virtual prices for CCD are the highest in the top group which leads to the conclusion that the contribution to efficiency per unit CCD is the biggest in the top group. This indicates that the quality of a unit CCD contributes positively to efficiency in this DEA setting. Between the middle and the low group no significant distinction is indicated.

➢ A similar conclusion holds for the input CCP. Again the top group has higher virtual price of CCP than the other two groups and therefore uses the best portion of CCP in relation to the output compared to the other two groups. Between the middle and the low group no significant distinction is found.

➢ The amount of fixed doctor relation has a significantly different effect on efficiency between the groups. The top group uses the existing long term doctor relations very efficiently in the sense that they can profit from such a relation regarding sales the most. This is indicated by the highest mean rank which the top group achieved.

Henceforth the fixed doctor relation contribute positively to efficiency. The two lower groups do not differ significantly in the category F/T.

➢ The most distinctive differences occur on the output side. The very low p-values between the top group and the two other groups underline that the target realization is an important driver of efficiency. Therefore the a high target realization increases efficiency.

Input/Output	Group	Group Average Weights	Mean Rank	z-value	doublesided p-value
Frequency	efficient 25%	5.72	25.6	0.73	0.4654
	middle 50%	0.33	22.5		
	efficient 25%	5.72	17.6	1.29	0.1971
	inefficient 25%	0.30	13.4		
	middle 50%	0.33	25	1.09	0.2757
	inefficient 25%	0.30	20.4		
CCD	efficient 25%	0.01498	33.3	3.43	0.0006
	middle 50%	0.00199	18.8		
	efficient 25%	0.01498	21.1	3.44	0.0006
	inefficient 25%	0.00179	9.9		
	middle 50%	0.00199	25.2	1.22	0.2225
	inefficient 25%	0.00179	20		
CCP	efficient 25%	0.00480	29.3	2.02	0.0434
	middle 50%	0.00251	20.7		
	efficient 25%	0.00480	19.7	2.59	0.0096
	inefficient 25%	0.00247	11.3		
	middle 50%	0.00251	25.5	1.48	0.1389
	inefficient 25%	0.00247	19.3		
F/T	efficient 25%	7.25	34.7	3.91	0.0001
	middle 50%	0.35	18.1		
	efficient 25%	7.25	20.2	2.92	0.0035
	inefficient 25%	0.36	10.8		
	middle 50%	0.35	21.5	-1.48	0.1389
	inefficient 25%	0.36	27.7		
TR	efficient 25%	5.13	38.3	5.2	<.0001
	middle 50%	0.78	16.3		
	efficient 25%	5.13	23	4.65	<.0001
	inefficient 25%	0.72	8		
	middle 50%	0.78	25.2	1.22	0.2225
	inefficient 25%	0.72	20		

Table 4.3.4-2: Results of the Mann Whitney U Test to identify reasons for efficieny

Summarizing the results above, one can conclude that the input frequency is used in the same intensity across the quartiles. The output TR seems to be very important for efficiency. The three inputs (CCD, CCP and F/T) all differ regarding the virtual prices between the top group and the lower two groups and, therefore, the virtual prices differ regarding the efficiency.

Groups	F	CCD	CCP	F/T	TR
efficient 25%	3.26	2.78	0.35	4.80	5.23
middle 50%	0.26	0.46	0.27	0.29	0.74
inefficient 25%	0.25	0.38	0.26	0.28	0.59

Table 4.3.4-3: Average virtual worth of the input or output category

Table 4.3.4-3 present the average virtual price times the average input and output amount in each of the categories. The table shows that especially in the middle and in the inefficient group the inputs CCP, F and F/T have a very low virtual worth in comparison to the categories CCD. Therefore, the three input categories with the lowest virtual worth seem to have a bigger improvement potential than the input CCD. On the output side, TR has to be increased. The biggest improvement potential lies within the inefficient 25%.

The conclusion from Table 4.3.4-3 is underlined by Table 4.3.4-4 which displays the overall optimization potential. The biggest optimizations on the input side are indicated with -21% for the input CCP, -14% points for the input F/T and -9% for F. The input CCD only has to be readjusted slightly. The optimal average target realization is calculated at 112%, which includes an increase from the current level by 16% points.

Input/Output	Actual Value	Target Value	Delta %
Ø F	81%	73%	-9%
CCD	13517	13021	-3.7%
CCP	6245	4907	-21%
Ø F/T	80%	66%	-14%
Ø TR	96%	112%	16%

Table 4.3.4-4: Comparison of current and optimal target values

In the next step the inter-temporal analysis is presented.

Inter-temporal Aspects

Figure 4.3.4-2 presents the development of the input and output categories from q1 2004 to q4 2006. The zero line for TR has been shifted to three for reasons of better illustration. The input CCD and CCP are divided by 100.

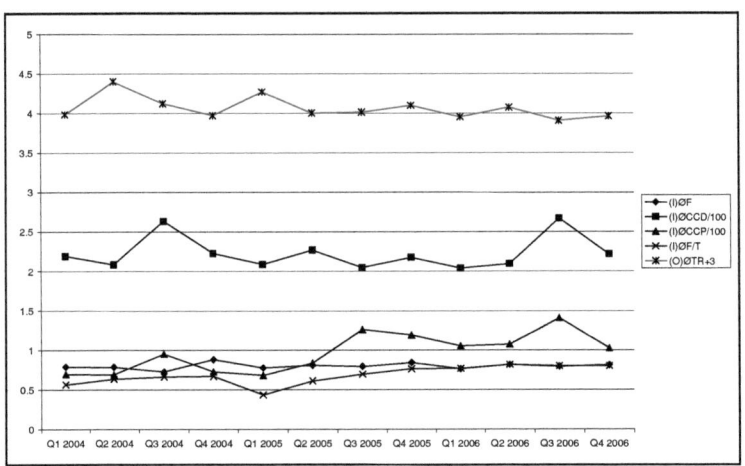

Figure 4.3.4-2: Development of average input and output values over *time (For reasons of graphical illustration: CCD and CCP divided by 100; TR plus 3)*

The output TR does not follow a clear trend. The target realization stays above 100% in average. The second quarter of 2004 and the first quarter 2005 are characterized by relatively high average target realizations (q2 2004: 140%; q1 2005: 127%). In addition the input side decreased in the above named two quarters. Therefore, the Malmquist Index should calculate high productivity increases. In q3 2004 the input side increases and the output decreases and, therefore, the MPI should be way below one.

These assumptions are supported by Table 4.3.4-5. The MPI for the quarters mentioned above underlines the assumptions stated above. The average MPI for the time periods displayed amounts to 1.06. Thus, the sales forces productivity increased, because the relation between effort invested and results achieved improved. The median has a similar tendency.

The standard deviation is the highest in the third row. This is partly due to an outlier in the data.

Malmquist	Average	Median	Max	Min	SD
q12004=>q22004	2.06	2.15	3.96	0.56	0.70
q22004=>q32004	0.72	0.66	1.71	0.37	0.27
q32004=>q42004	0.92	0.77	7.29	0.38	0.89
q42004=>q12005	1.91	1.88	3.97	0.20	0.75
q12005=>q22005	0.70	0.66	1.52	0.37	0.27
q22005=>q32005	0.93	0.91	1.51	0.21	0.26
q32005=>q42005	1.04	0.97	1.95	0.60	0.29
q42005=>q12006	0.97	0.96	1.53	0.45	0.23
q12006=>q22006	1.12	1.11	2.13	0.50	0.28
q22006=>q32006	0.80	0.75	2.31	0.35	0.31
q32006=>q42006	1.26	1.21	2.03	0.33	0.33

Table 4.3.4-5: Average productivity development described by the overall MPI

The efficiency development of the sales force is displayed below in Table 4.3.4-6 and indicates that in this DEA version the sales force has got great improvement potential. The maximum average score achieved is 0.77 in q3 2005 and q1 2006. The lowest score attained is 0.49 in q1 2004. As stated in the other versions the average efficiency scores still leave room for upward improvements for the sales force. For more sales success the management has to bring the sales force on an upward trend with a lower variance of the average efficiency scores by taking into account the outcomes of the analysis of the individual sales reps.

Quarters	Ø Efficiency
q1 2004	0.49
q2 2004	0.62
q3 2004	0.66
q4 2004	0.58
q1 2005	0.68
q2 2005	0.60
q3 2005	0.77
q4 2005	0.74
q1 2006	0.77
q2 2006	0.73
q3 2006	0.66
q4 2006	0.76

Table 4.3.4-6 Development of Ø efficiency

Due to the fact that the conclusions and effects on the individual level in this DEA version differ from the other DEA versions, the individual optimization possibilities will be regarded next.

Benchmarking of individual sales reps

Figure 4.3.4-3 displays the results for SR 4 who is ranked number one and achieves an efficiency score of 118%. With six times mentioned in the reference sets of inefficient sales reps SR4 reached rank 5 regarding the frequency. The impact value of 2.1 corresponds to rank 5 as well. The MPI of SR4 accounts to 1.17 and, therefore, the productivity of SR4 increases from quarter to quarter. The efficiency development reveals a nice upward trend, reaching the efficiency status in the fourth quarter of 2006.

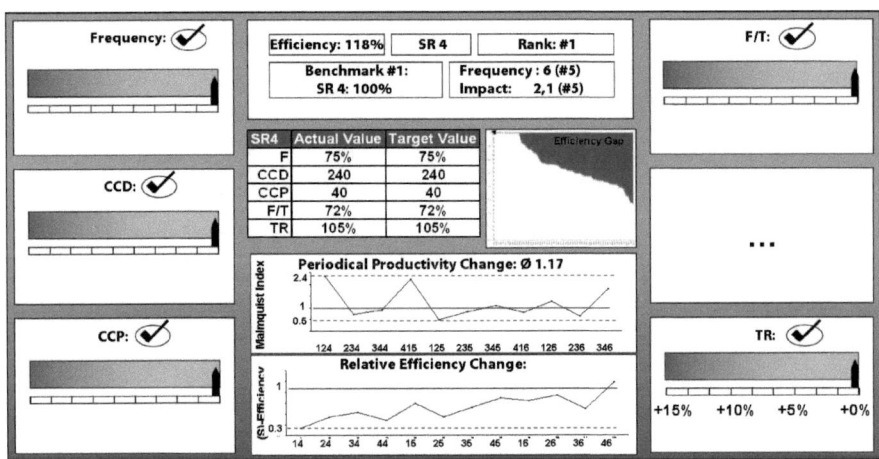

Figure 4.3.4-3: KPI-Cockpit for SR 4 (F, CCD, CCP, F/T – TR)

In comparison to the version with F, CCD, CCP, F/T as inputs and Q and CI as outputs, sales rep 4 is still very efficient but is not mentioned as a benchmark partner as often, due to a transformation system of inputs to outputs, which is obviously not according to the "main stream".

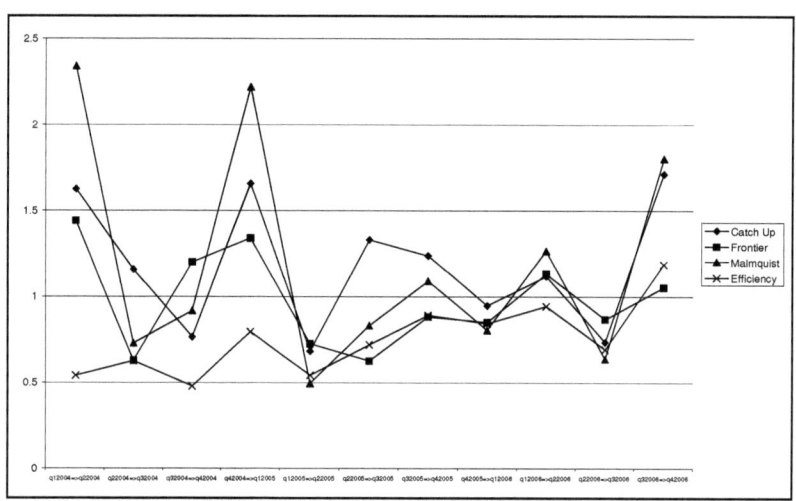

Figure 4.3.4-4: Decomposition of the MPI and the efficiency development of SR4

The decomposition of the MPI is displayed in Figure 4.3.4-4. The average frontier shift amounts to 0.99 on average, indicating that the total factor productivity of the benchmark partners of SR4 is decreasing. The CU is above one most of the time with an average value of 1.13. Hence, the efficiency of SR4 has increased together with total factor productivity.

SR 28 in the figure below is ranked number #35 and reached an efficiency score of 0.72. The most important benchmark partners are SR59 with 76% and SR 54 with 24%. The inputs F, CCP and F/T need improvement. The output target realization should be increased by 21% points. The biggest contribution to inefficiency stems from the output side, which is nearly two times bigger than the contribution to inefficiency on the input side. This fact highlights that the biggest improvements regarding efficiency can be achieved only by increasing the output side.

The MPI of SR 28 increases in average from year to year and efficiency is rising. Regarding these facts SR 28 is undergoing a positive development.

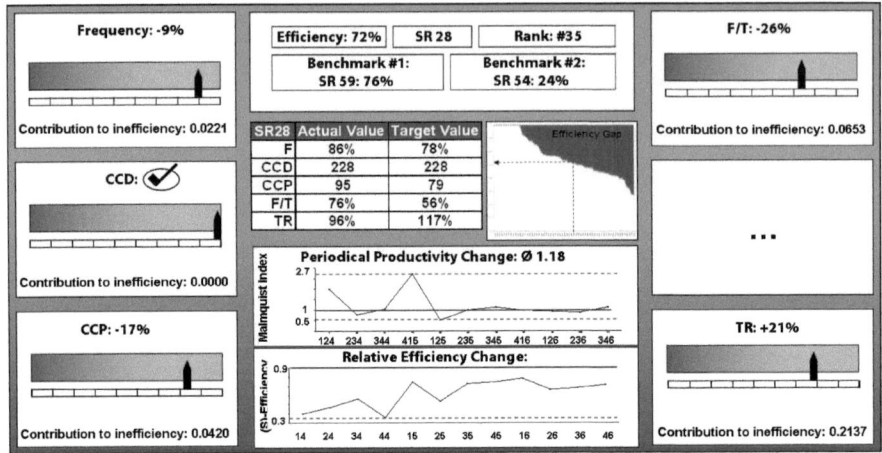

Figure 4.3.4-5: KPI-Cockpit for SR 28 (F, CCD, CCP, F/T – TR)

Figure 4.3.4-6 depicts that the variances of the CU, the frontier shift and the MPI. Due to the upward-trend in the efficiency from 0.3 to about 0.7 the average CU is greater than one. Therefore, SR28 is improving the sales process faster than its benchmark partners. The benchmark partners in turn are experiencing an average increase in productivity, which is indicated by a frontier shift above one. Henceforth the total factor productivity is increasing as well as does the relative efficiency score.

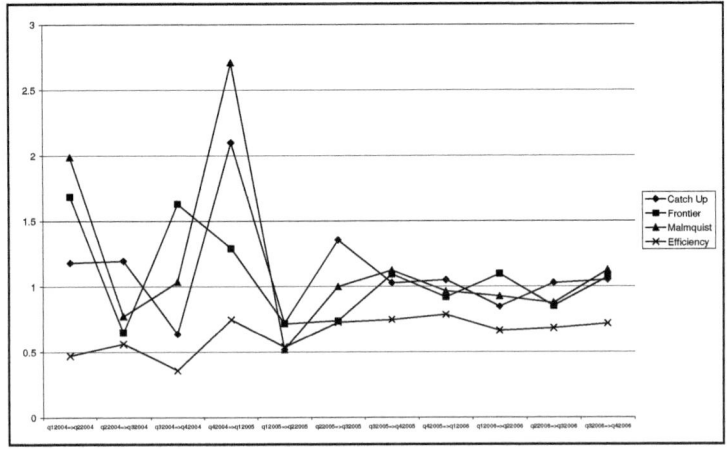

Figure 4.3.4-6: Decomposition of the MPI and the efficiency development of SR28

Finally, SR 42 shall be analysed regarding the influences on efficiency aspects, caused by a changed DEA setting. As in the previous chapter with SOM as output SR 42 is assigned a higher efficiency score due to the inclusion of TR as output. The efficiency score calculates at 61%, which is much better than in the previous calculations. The main benchmark partners are SR54 (66%) and SR4 (13%). The input F should be reduced by 30% and the output TR should be increased by 50%. The main contribution to inefficiency stems from the output side. The input side has only a minor effect on the efficiency score of q4 2006.

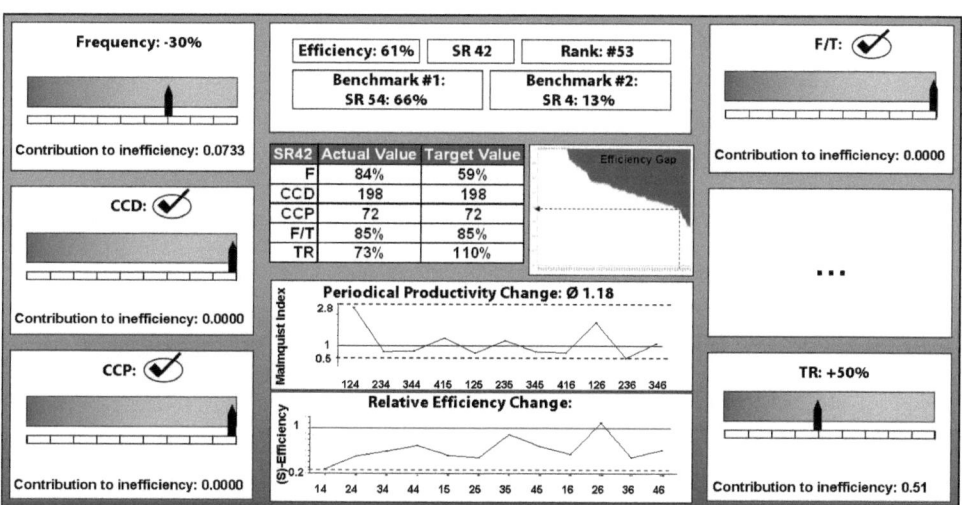

Figure 4.3.4-7: KPI-Cockpit for SR 42 (F, CCD, CCP, F/T – SOM)

In this setting the average MPI calculates at 1.18 and the efficiency score is increasing slightly from about 0.3 to 0.6 but with big variances. Therefore, SR 42 has to undertake strong improvements to reach the efficiency frontier.

The decomposition of the MPI shows the following:
The CU is greater than one in average (1.18), which reflects the fact that efficiency is rising over time. The frontier shift in average keeps to one and therefore the efficiency frontier in the projection region does not really move. Due to the fact that the efficiency frontier did not move the main driver of the productivity increase can be found within the production process of SR 42. SR 42 was able to transform his inputs in to increasing amounts of output over the twelve

quarters. However this happened on a very low scale which reflects in the slow efficiency increase of SR42.

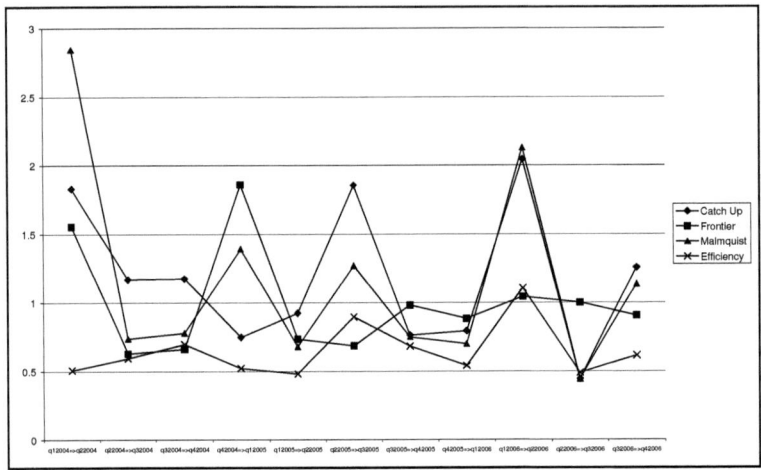

Figure 4.3.4-8: Decomposition of the MPI and the efficiency development of SR42

4.3.5 SBM Model Version 5 (F, CCD, F/T, TR)

The following DEA version takes into account TR as the single output and F, CCD and F/T as inputs.

The Efficiency Gap

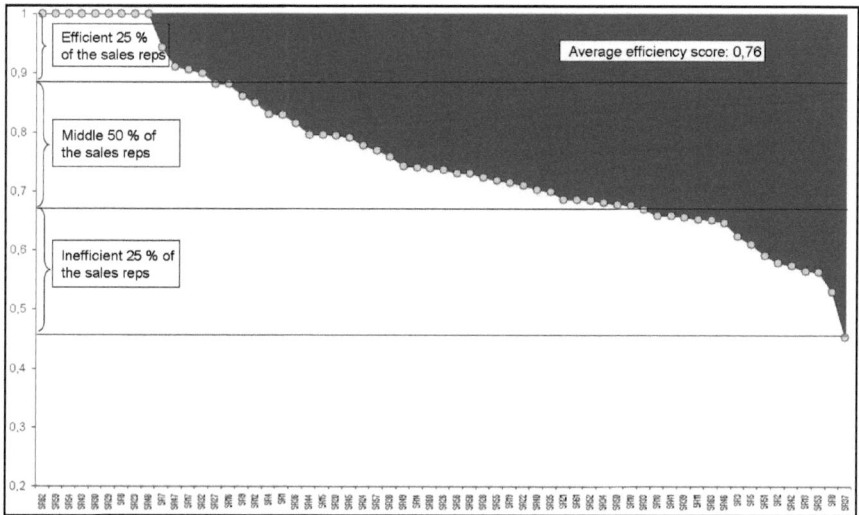

Figure 4.3.5-1: Illustration of the Efficiency Gap and of the three efficiency groups

The efficiency gap ranges from 1 to 0.46. The average efficiency score calculates at 0.76. Nine sales reps reach an efficient status. Compared to previous DEA settings the smaller number of efficient sales rep is due to the fact that the dimensions of this DEA setting are reduced to four.

Table 4.3.5-1 depicts the average efficiency scores for the groups calculated by applying the different DEA models using F, CCD, F/T as inputs and TR as output. The table shows that the SBM measure is the strictest, followed by the CCR model. In contrast to most of the other

DEA settings the efficient group never reaches 100% efficiency in average, which is due to the reduced number of dimensions.

F,CCD, F/T – TR Group	Average SBM-NO-V Efficiency	Average BCC-O Efficiency	Average CCR-O Efficiency
Efficient 25%	96%	97%	97%
Middle 50%	75%	80%	79%
Inefficient 25%	60%	66%	63%

Table 4.3.5-1: Comparison of average efficiency scores

Table 4.3.5-2 seeks to identify the reasons for a high efficiency score regarding the output and input categories.

- Concerning the input F no significant difference on a level $p \leq 5\%$ is detected. On a significance level of $p \leq 10\%$ it can be stated that there is a difference in F between the efficient and middle group in the sense that the efficient group has a higher average virtual price for F. Hence, in this setting, the efficient group uses the input frequency more intensively than the middle group.

- Looking at the input CCD significant ($p \leq 5\%$) differences between the efficient 25% and the middle group and between the efficient 25% and the inefficient 25% occur. Once again this detail points out that the efficient group is better at using the input CCD compared to the others in reaching their targets.

- The higher the virtual weight of the input F/T, so better is the group efficiency. The top group uses the existing long term doctor relations very efficiently in the sense that they profit the most from such a relation regarding sales. This is indicated by the highest mean rank which the top group achieved. Henceforth fixed doctor relations contribute to efficiency but on a different scale for each group. The two inferior groups do not differ significantly in the category F/T.

- The most distinctive differences occur on the output side. The very low p-values between the top group and the other two groups underline that the target realization is an important driver of efficiency. Therefore, a high target realization increases efficiency.

Input/Output	Group	Group Average Weights	Mean Rank	z-value	doublesided p-value
Frequency	efficient 25%	2.59	28.3	1.68	0.093
	middle 50%	0.41	21.2		
	efficient 25%	2.59	18.1	1.58	0.1141
	inefficient 25%	0.40	12.9		
	middle 50%	0.41	23.7	0.13	0.8966
	inefficient 25%	0.40	23.1		
CCD	efficient 25%	0.00402	30.1	2.3	0.0214
	middle 50%	0.00202	20.3		
	efficient 25%	0.00402	19.7	2.57	0.0102
	inefficient 25%	0.00171	11.3		
	middle 50%	0.00202	25.3	1.27	0.2041
	inefficient 25%	0.00171	19.9		
F/T	efficient 25%	3.57528	33.8	3.61	0.0003
	middle 50%	0.41707	18.5		
	efficient 25%	3.57528	20.7	3.24	0.0012
	inefficient 25%	0.40230	10.3		
	middle 50%	0.41707	23.5	0	1
	inefficient 25%	0.40230	23.5		
TR	efficient 25%	1.00	37.1	4.76	<.0001
	middle 50%	0.78	16.9		
	efficient 25%	1.00	23	4.65	<.0001
	inefficient 25%	0.73	8		
	middle 50%	0.78	25.4	1.38	0.1676
	inefficient 25%	0.73	19.5		

Table 4.3.5-2: Results of the Mann Whitney U Test to identify sources of efficiency

Summarizing the results above, it can be conclude that the input frequency is not so important for the achievement of a high efficiency score in this setting. The output TR seems to be very important for efficiency. The two inputs (CCD, and F/T) both differ regarding the virtual prices between the top group and the poorer two groups and, therefore, all have an influence on the average efficiency scores.

Table 4.3.5-3 presents the average virtual price times the average input and output amount in each of the categories. The table shows that in the middle and in the inefficient group, particularly the inputs F and F/T have a lower virtual worth in comparison to the category

CCD. Therefore the two input categories with the lowest virtual worth seem to have a greater improvement potential than the input CCD. On the output side TR has to be increased. Here the greatest improvement potential lies within the inefficient 25%.

Groups	F	CCD	F/T	TR
efficient 25%	1.68	0.79	2.20	1.06
middle 50%	0.34	0.43	0.34	0.76
inefficient 25%	0.34	0.39	0.33	0.60

Table 4.3.5-3: Average virtual worth of the input or output category

The results of Table 4.3.5-3 is confirmed by Table 4.3.5-4 which displays the overall optimization potential. The greatest optimizations on the input side are indicated with -21% for the input F/T and -15% for F. The input CCD only has to be readjusted slightly. The optimal average target realization is calculated at 112%, which includes an increase from the current level by 16% points.

Input/Output	Actual Value	Target Value	Delta %
Ø F	81%	69%	-15%
CCD	13517	12951	-4%
Ø F/T	80%	63%	-21%
Ø TR	96%	110%	15%

Table 4.3.5-4: Comparison of current and optimal target values

In the following the inter-temporal analysis is presented.

Inter-temporal Aspects

Figure 4.3.5-2 presents the development of the input and output categories from q1 2004 to q4 2006. As before, the zero line for TR has been shifted to three for reasons of better illustration. The input CCD is divided by 100.

As described in the previous chapter the output TR does not follow a clear trend. The target realization stays above 100% in average. The second quarter 2004 and the first quarter 2005 are characterized by relatively high average target realizations (q2 2004: 140%; q1 2005: 127%). In addition, the input side decreased in the two quarters named above. Therefore, the Malmquist Index should calculate high productivity increases. In q3 2004 the input side increases and the output decreases and, therefore, the MPI should be way below one. The input CCP is not included.

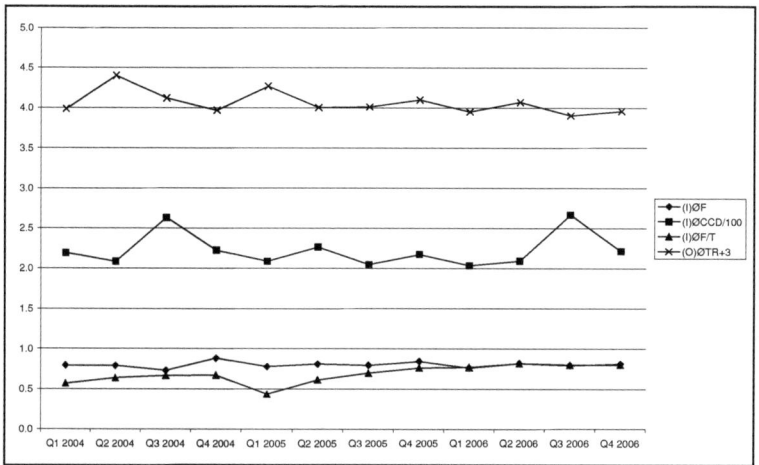

Figure 4.3.5-2: Development of average input and output values over *time (For reasons of graphical illustration: CCD divided by 100; TR plus 3)*

These assumptions are supported by Table 4.3.5-5. The MPI for the quarters mentioned above underlines the assumptions stated before. The average MPI for the time periods displayed amounts to 1.06. Thus the sales forces productivity increased because the relation between effort invested and results achieved improved. The median has a similar tendency. The standard deviation is the highest in the third row. This is partly due to an outlier in the data.

The efficiency development of the sales force is displayed below and indicates that the sales force still has great improvement potential. The maximum average score achieved is 0.78 in q4 2005. The lowest score attained is 0.51 in q1 2004. As stated in the other versions, the average efficiency scores still leave room for upward improvements for the sales force.

Malmquist	Average	Median	Max	Min	SD
q12004=>q22004	1.97	2.02	3.64	0.67	0.65
q22004=>q32004	0.77	0.73	1.73	0.34	0.28
q32004=>q42004	0.80	0.75	3.22	0.40	0.38
q42004=>q12005	1.73	1.70	3.68	0.43	0.61
q12005=>q22005	0.74	0.71	1.77	0.39	0.26
q22005=>q32005	1.05	1.03	1.71	0.28	0.26
q32005=>q42005	1.02	0.95	1.82	0.64	0.27
q42005=>q12006	0.92	0.90	1.60	0.42	0.21
q12006=>q22006	1.13	1.10	2.23	0.47	0.28
q22006=>q32006	0.84	0.79	2.17	0.40	0.28
q32006=>q42006	1.15	1.13	2.07	0.36	0.27

Table 4.3.5-5: Development of the MPI over time

In this DEA setting, however, the average efficiency as depicted in Table 4.3.5-6 of the sales force seems to be on an upward trend but reached a plateau in 2006. Therefore, the sales management should undertake an in depth analysis of the single sales reps.

Quarter	Ø Efficiency
q1 2004	0.51
q2 2004	0.58
q3 2004	0.62
q4 2004	0.66
q1 2005	0.67
q2 2005	0.62
q3 2005	0.76
q4 2005	0.78
q1 2006	0.76
q2 2006	0.75
q3 2006	0.70
q4 2006	0.76

Table 4.3.5-6: Development of Ø efficiency

In the next section the individual sales reps will be highlighted and improvement opportunities will be revealed.

Benchmarking of individual sales reps

Figure 4.3.5-3 displays the results for SR 4, who is ranked #18 and achieves an efficiency score of 83%. Hence SR 4 failed to reach an efficient status. This fact is very interesting because the present DEA setting is the only one where SR 4 fails to be efficient.

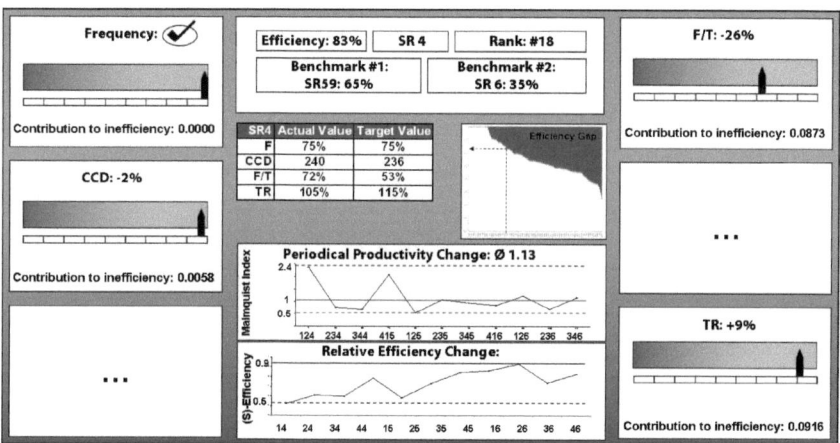

Figure 4.3.5-3: KPI-Cockpit for SR 4 (F, CCD, CCP, F/T – TR)

Because of the exclusion of CCP, SR 4 fell back so far that an efficient status could not be reached anymore. The conclusion, drawn in chapter 4.3.2 that the input CCP is very important for SR 4 regarding the efficiency score, is confirmed.

The input F is green. CCD needs slight upgrading and the input F/T has to be improved by -26%. This finding sheds light on the fact that SR4 could achieve at least the same results with less long term doctor relations *in this DEA version*. The target realization should increase by 9%. Another interesting fact is that, in this setting the biggest contribution to inefficiency stems from the input side. Hence the sum of the contributions to inefficiency of the input side is slightly higher than that of the output side. Therefore, SR4 may work on the input side first in order to improve his efficiency.

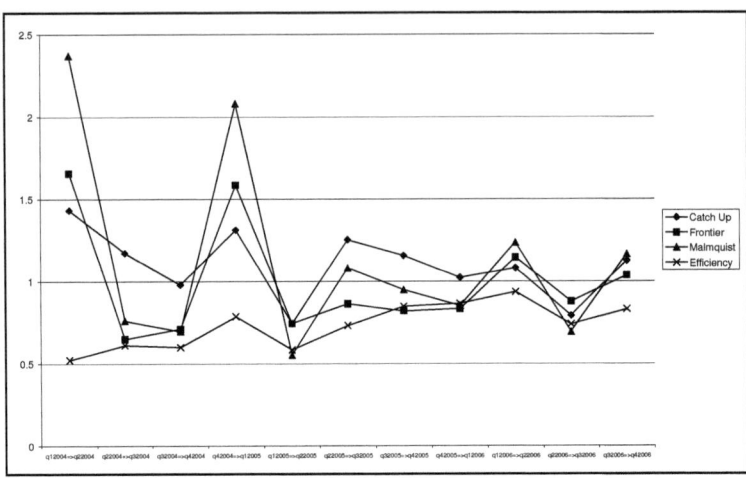

Figure 4.3.5-4: Decomposition of the MPI and the efficiency development of SR4

The decomposition of the MPI is displayed in Figure 4.3.5-4. The average frontier shift amounts to 0.99 indicating that the total factor productivity of the benchmark partners of SR4 was decreasing. The CU is above one most of the time with an average value of 1.13. This in turn indicates that SR4 is improving the efficiency of the production process.

SR 28 is ranked number 34 and reached an efficiency score of 0.72. The most important benchmark partners are SR59 with 80% and SR 29 with 20%. The inputs F and F/T need improvement. The output target realization should be increased by 20% points. The biggest contribution to inefficiency stems from the output side. This fact highlights that the biggest improvements regarding efficiency can be achieved by increasing output. The exclusion of the input CCP has very little impact on SR28. This indicates that CCP is not so important concerning the efficiency score for SR28.

The MPI of SR 28 increases with an average rate of 1.11. In addition, the efficiency development of SR 28 is showing an upward trend. Regarding these facts SR 28 appears to experience a fine development.

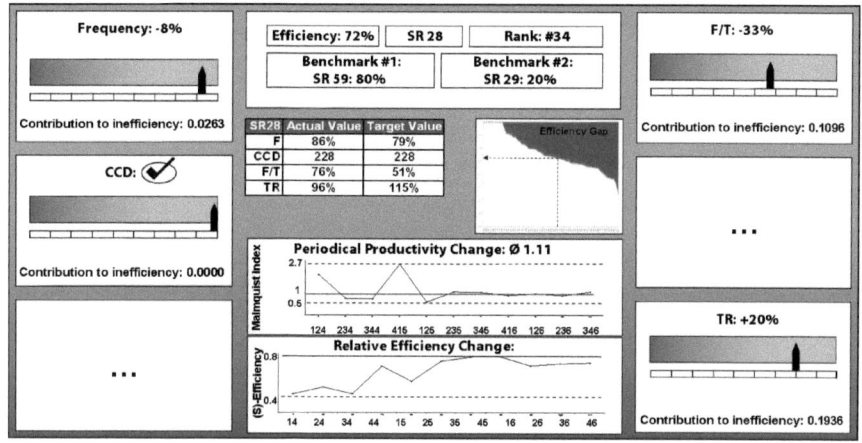

Figure 4.3.5-5: KPI-Cockpit for SR 28 (F, CCD, F/T – TR)

Figure 4.3.5-6 shows the variances of the CU, the frontier shift and the MPI. Due to the upward-trend in the efficiency from 0.5 to about 0.75, the average CU is greater than one. Therefore, SR28 is improving the sales process faster than its benchmark partners. The benchmark partners in turn are experiencing an average increase in productivity, which is indicated by a frontier shift above one. Hence, the total factor productivity is increasing, indicated by an average MPI above one. Therefore the relative efficiency score increases as well. Interestingly, the volatility of the curves decreases as time passes. Based on this DEA version, it can be assumed that SR28 may have been a new employee at the beginning of 2004 and than gained experience which improved the sales results.

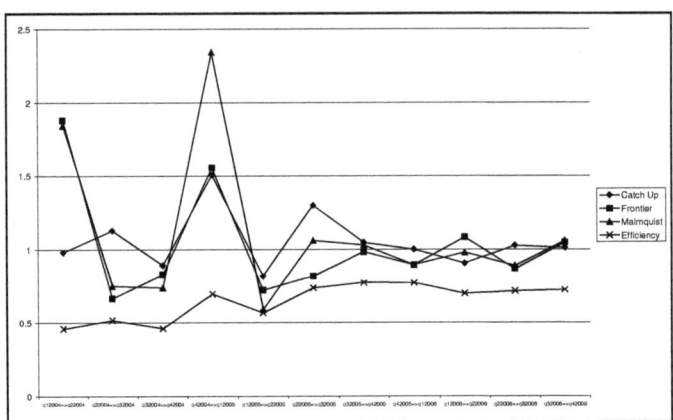

Figure 4.3.5-6: Decomposition of the Malmquistindex and development of relative efficiency

The last individual analysis of the impact of a changed DEA setting on efficiency can be seen in SR 42 (see Figure 4.3.5-7) The efficiency score calculates at 0.57, which is much better than in the calculations with Q and CI as output but weaker than the calculation with CCP as additional input and TR as output (see chapter 4.3.4).

Hence, the exclusion of CCP as input has a negative effect on the efficiency score of SR42 *in this setting*.

The main benchmark partners are SR29 (70%) and SR59 (30%). The input F should be reduced by 32% and the output TR should be increased by 44%. The main contribution to inefficiency stems from the output side. The input side has only a minor effect on the efficiency score of q4 2006 and, therefore, it would be advisable to increase his target realization first before improving the input side.

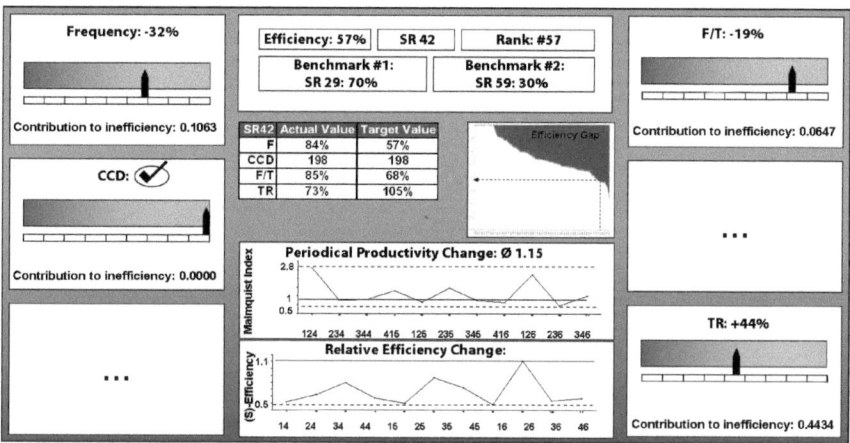

Figure 4.3.5-7: KPI-Cockpit for SR 42 (F, CCD, CCP, F/T – SOM)

In this setting the average MPI calculates at 1.15 and the efficiency score is hovering around 0.65 with a relatively high variance. Therefore, no clear trend with reference to efficiency is detected.

The decomposition of the MPI shows the following (see Figure 4.3.5-8):
The CU is greater than one in average (1.15). Nevertheless, this finding does not support the statement that the efficiency of SR42 increased over time. The CU is greater than one due to high peaks in the graph which level out the average score. The development of the efficiency frontier in the projection region of SR42 is fairly poor and stays beneath one from the second quarter of 2005 onwards. Unfortunately, SR42 fails to reach a sustainable catch up path.

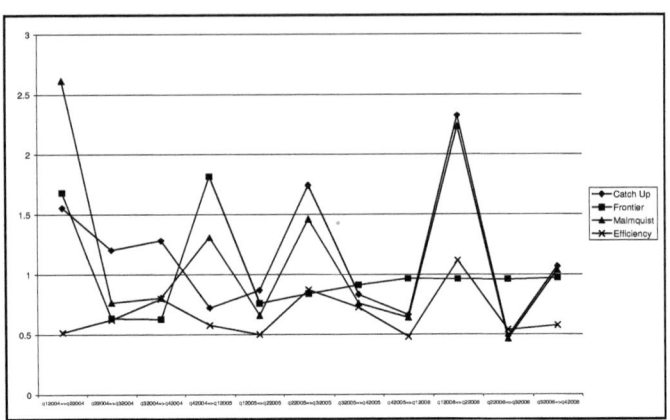

Figure 4.3.5-8: Decomposition of the Malmquistindex and efficiency development for SR42

Instead the catch up process shows big disruptions by overshooting one and crashing way beneath one. In the last six quarters SR42 is experiencing a strong side movement regarding efficiency. SR42 did not improve very much and remained on a same efficiency and productivity level. Such a development is unfavourable and should be closely analysed. As concluded before, this DEA version shows the need for SR42 to improve greatly.

4.3.6 Summary of the SBM DEA model

In this section the results of the SBM model are summarized. First the efficiency gaps of the different SBM DEA settings are presented.

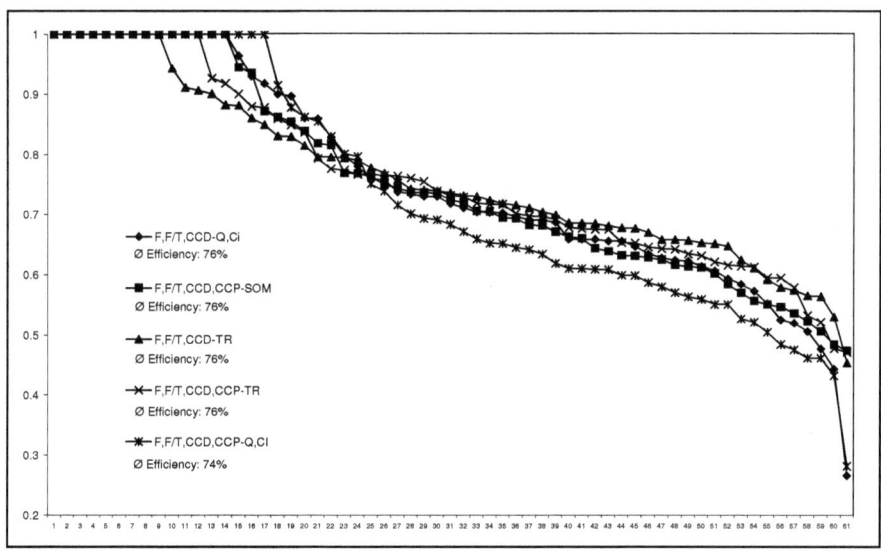

Figure 4.3.6-1: Comparison of the different efficiency gaps

Regarding the average efficiency score of the sample the DEA setting wit F, F/T, CCD, CCP as inputs and Q and CI as outputs is the strictest efficiency measure (line with stars). However, the star line begins with depicting most of the sales reps as efficient but after leaving the efficient level, it drops down steeply and reveals itself as the line with the lowest efficiency scores. The high number of efficient units is due to the fact that the setting, resulting in the star line, is the only one taking six dimensions into account.

This statement is confirmed by the triangle line which identifies the smallest amount of sales reps as efficient due to the reduction of the dimensions to four.

It is worth mentioning that the average efficiency score of four models calculates at 0.76, no matter which DEA setting is used. The other model with an 0.74 average efficiency score, reaches very closely to the efficiency score of 0.76. Therefore, the "true" efficiency score of the sales force probably lies somewhere in the middle of the seventies when using the SBM model. Hence an upward potential regarding efficiency of a maximum of about 25% is possible. This upward potential can be transformed into sales forecasts which are presented in the upcoming paragraphs (see Table 4.3.6-9).

Next, Figure 4.3.6-2 displays the average efficiency development of the different SBM DEA settings. The figure shows that, as time passes, the differences between the efficiency scores diminish. At the beginning of the time interval it is obvious that those settings which include the output Q achieve better efficiency scores.

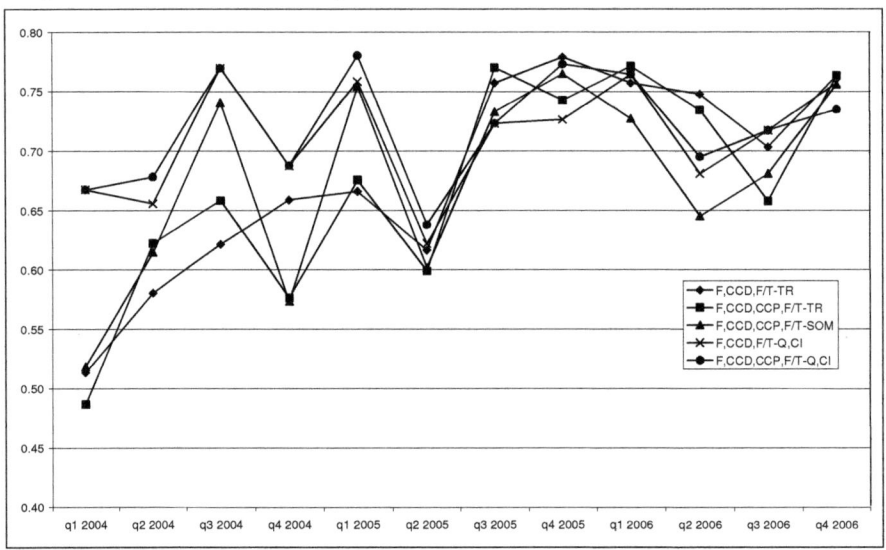

Figure 4.3.6-2: Efficiency developments over time for the different DEA settings

The DEA settings which exclude Q as output are fairly weak concerning the average efficiency score. To confirm this finding the Mann Whitney U Test was applied to the data, resulting in Table 4.3.6-1 which confirms that the differences in the average efficiency scores for q1 2004 are not calculated randomly. Hence, the inclusion of Q into the analysis has a positive effect on efficiency. Those sales reps, with bad efficiency scores in the cases where Q is excluded could compensate a good deal of the inefficiency by the inclusion of Q, with regards to version 3 (SOM as output).

	Quarter 1 2004			
DEA setting	average efficiency score	mean rank	z-value	double sided p-value
F,CCD,CCP,F/T-TR	0.49	47.2	4.46	<.0001
F,CCD,CCP,F/T-Q,CI	0.67	75.8		
F,CCD,CCP,F/T-SOM	0.52	49.9	3.62	0.0003
F,CCD,CCP,F/T-Q,CI	0.67	73.1		
F,CCD,F/T-TR	0.51	49.6	3.72	0.0002
F,CCD,CCP,F/T-Q,CI	0.67	73.4		

Table 4.3.6-1: Significance of differences in the efficiency scores

Regarding the fact that the input structure is (almost) the same in Table 4.3.6-1, the only explanation for the differences in the efficiency scores is that at the beginning of the interval sales reps with a low efficiency (poor SOM or TR) in tendency sold higher absolute amounts of Q, compared to those sales reps with a high SOM or TR. Therefore, after the inclusion of Q into the analysis, sales reps with low SOM or TR experienced an "upgrade" which increased the overall efficiency score. The increase in efficiency scores is due to the fact that the differences between sales reps on the output side are not so determent anymore. If the characteristic of the output side would not have changed by the inclusion of Q into the analysis, the average efficiency score would have not changed. To confirm this assumption the attention is drawn to Table 4.3.6-2.

	Quarter 1 2004			
(F,CCD,CCP,F/T-SOM) Groups	Ø Q/SOM	Mean Rank	Z-Value	Double sided P-Value
efficient 25%	4.90	17.3	-2.18	0.0293
middle 50%	5.83	26.5		
efficient 25%	4.90	11.7	-2.36	0.0183
inefficient 25%	6.22	19.3		
middle 50%	5.83	22.6	0.63	0.5287
inefficient 25%	6.22	25.3		

Table 4.3.6-2: Evidence for the positive effect of Q on efficiency

The table depicts version 3 with SOM as output for the first quarter 2004. A main driver of efficiency in this version is the market share, similar as described in chapter 4.3.3 for the fourth quarter 2006. For each of the three groups the relation between Q and SOM was calculated. The relation between Q and SOM should be higher, the lower the efficiency score is in the DEA setting with only SOM as output. This would reveal that inefficient sales reps (with low market share) sold relatively much insulin. In that case the inclusion of Q into the analysis would compensate lower SOM values and, thus, lead to increased average efficiency. This tendency is confirmed by Table 4.3.6-2 which highlights that the efficient 25% in the DEA setting with SOM as output have a lower relation between Q and SOM than the other two groups (level of significance: $p \leq 5\%$). The sales reps with weak efficiency in the version with only SOM as output could catch up. Therefore the average efficiency increased through the inclusion of Q into the analysis.

These differences regarding the achieved average efficiency score between the DEA settings with and without Q as output remain until the first quarter 2005 (see Figure 4.3.6-2). The managerial implication of this finding is that the best sales reps (from an efficiency point of view) were working in the markets with lower sales potential and the weak sales reps in the markets with higher sales potential. To increase sales success the sales reps should have been reallocated.

From the second quarter 2005 onwards such a compensating effect of Q on the efficiency scores cannot be identified anymore as Table 4.3.6-3 displays.

(F,CCD,CCP,F/T-SOM) Groups	Quarter 2 2005			Double sided
	Ø Q/SOM	Mean Rank	Z-Value	P-Value
efficient 25%	13.17	25.50	0.70	0.48
middle 50%	13.01	22.50		
efficient 25%	13.17	17.50	1.24	0.22
inefficient 25%	12.20	13.50		
middle 50%	13.01	24.90	0.98	0.33
inefficient 25%	12.20	20.70		

Table 4.3.6-3: The difference of Q/SOM between the quartiles disappears.

The mean ranks of the groups as well as the average relation between Q and SOM of the groups are pretty close to each other. This occurrence could have been caused by a rearrangement of territories so that the efficient sales reps could achieve high market shares in markets with high sales potential.

The exclusion of the input CCP has no big influence on the efficiency results of the DEA setting with Q and CI as outputs. This statement can be confirmed by a close look at Figure 4.3.6-2. The two lines with crosses and circles move quite close together which indicates that the difference in the average efficiency score of the sample caused by the exclusion of CCP is limited.

A similar conclusion holds for the DEA settings with TR as output. The exclusion of CCP only has limited effects on the efficiency scores as well but, however, these limited effects are a bit more pronounced especially in the fourth quarter 2004.

The summaries for the sales reps 4, 28 and 42 are presented in Table 4.3.6-4, Table 4.3.6-5 and Table 4.3.6-6. The percentage values in the input and output lines are the percentage decreases (for inputs) and increases (for outputs) according to the status quo. The benchmark lines display the impact of the different efficient SRs as mentoring partner for the evaluated sales rep in the specific setting. The last line depicts the efficiency score of the evaluated sales rep in each of the DEA variants. The columns show the different DEA settings.

SR 4		(1)F,F/T,CCD,CCP-Q,CI	(2)F,F/T,CCD-Q,CI	(3)F,F/T,CCD,CCP-SOM	(4)F,F/T,CCD,CCP-TR	(5)F,F/T,CCD-TR
Inputs	F	0.00%	0.00%	0.00%	0.00%	0.00%
	CCD	0.00%	0.00%	0.00%	0.00%	-1.76%
	CCP	0.00%	~	0.00%	0.00%	~
	F/T	0.00%	0.00%	0.00%	0.00%	-26.20%
Outputs	Q	0.00%	0.00%	~	~	~
	CI	0.00%	0.00%	~	~	~
	TR	~	~	~	0.00%	9.16%
	SOM	~	~	0.00%	~	~
Benchmarks	SR6	~	~	~	~	0.35
	SR59	~	~	~	~	0.65
Efficiency		129%	104%	118%	118%	83%

Table 4.3.6-4: Summary of SR4

Sales rep 4 in Table 4.3.6-4 is inefficient only in the setting (5) with F, F/T, CCD as inputs and TR as output. Therefore only in this setting benchmark partners are assigned to SR 4 and an output expansion of 9.16% is calculated. Due to the assumption of VRS the benchmark weights add up to one and henceforth they can be interpreted as impact of a mentor on a sales rep expressed in percent.

Furthermore the exclusion of CCP has got a negative effect on the efficiency score. In addition the change from Q and CI as outputs to the single output TR has a negative effect on efficiency as well. The output SOM seems to have a similar effect on the efficiency of SR4 as the output TR (compare (4) with (3)).

Henceforth, the output TR and SOM seem to be not advantageous for SR4. This sales rep is strong when it comes to absolute amounts of Q sold and the inclusion of the CCP measure, which is used very efficiently. However, in DEA versions (1) to (3) the sales rep is efficient and the statement concerning the effects of inputs and outputs on efficiency only effect "Super" efficiency and do not change the overall efficient status of the sales rep. The overall efficient status is only changed in DEA version (5) where two disadvantages hit SR 4 at the same time, the exclusion of CCP, Q and CI and the inclusion of TR as output, and thus the efficiency score decreases below one.

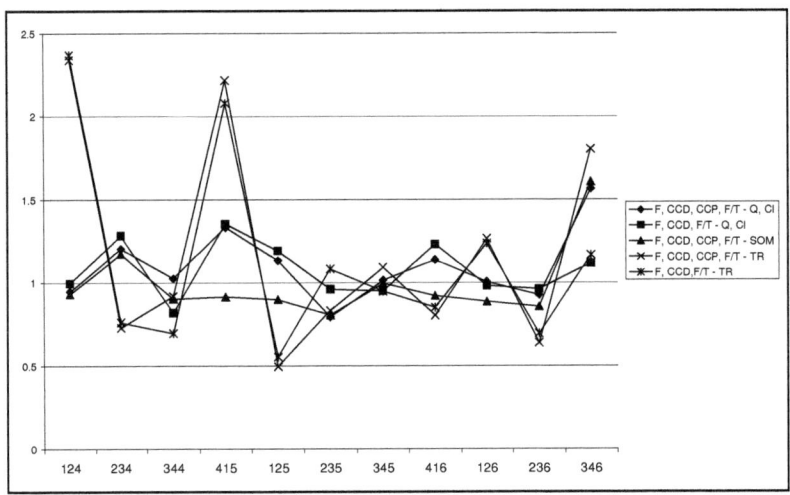

Figure 4.3.6-3: Development of the MPI for the different DEA versions for SR4

Figure 4.3.6-3 displays the different MPIs of SR4 for each of the SBM DEA versions. The versions excluding CCP as inputs moved closely with the versions including CCP. Hence the exclusion or inclusion of CCP did not have a big impact on the MPI and therefore the reasons for shifts in productivity do not have their origin in the input CCP. Only in the last quarter of 2006 the input CCP contributes significantly positively to the MPI. This confirms the findings from chapter 4.3.1 and 4.3.4, that SR4 was very efficient in the use of CCP in the fourth quarter 2006 SR4.

The reasons for different developments of the MPI therefore can be found on the output side rather. There are great differences depending on the outputs chosen for the analysis. If the output SOM is included, the MPI mainly remains below one and hence the total factor productivity decreases. This goes in line with the overall market condition presented at the beginning of chapter 3. If the outputs Q and CI are included the MPI of SR4 is very volatile in contrast to the versions including TR as output which are less volatile. An explanation could be detected in the definition of TR. TR accounts for past market developments and the targets for a sales rep are set with respect to this development. The output Q, for instance, always reflects the market development unadjusted and therefore the high volatility occurs.

SR 28 is inefficient in every SBM DEA version. The efficiency scores of SR 28 range between 0.73 (2) and 0.67 (1). The input F has to be adjusted in every version. The biggest adjustment of -40.7% has to be undertaken in version (3) whereas the other versions only recommend moderate adjustments with a maximum of -8.8%. The reason for the high adjustment of F is that in version (3) SR28 has only SR6 as benchmark partner. Therefore the optimum of SR 28 in version (3) is exactly equal to the input and output vector of SR6 which has a frequency 40.7% lower than that of SR28 in the status quo.

The only DEA version where the input CCD is adjusted is (2). The adjustment of CCD is very moderate and accounts to -10% only in version (2) and hence SR28 is more or less efficient in the use of CCD.

The input CCP has to be adjusted in each version it is implied in. Interestingly the highest adjustment of CCP is in version (1) where SR 4 is the main benchmark partner. This underlines the statement that SR4 is very efficient in the use of CCP.

Generally speaking SR28 has quite a high adjustment needs in the input category CCP. The extent of the adjustments of the input F/T differs distinctively between the versions. In version (5) F/T has to be reduced by as much as 33% and in version (1) and (3) by about 8%. These differences result from the different benchmark partners SR28 is assigned in the different versions.

The recommendations for Q and CI are almost the same in version (1) and (2) and therefore the exclusion of CCP has almost no influence on the adjustment needs of Q and CI for SR28, although it has a negative influence on the specific efficiency score. This indicates that SR28 is not so good in the use of CCP compared to the rest of the sample.

The optimal projections for TR and SOM are similar especially for the versions including CCP as input.

Regarding the benchmark partner a remarkable fact is that in version (3) SR6 is the only benchmark. In all other versions there are two benchmarking partners, of which one is about three times as important as the other.

SR28		(1)F,F/T,CCD,CCP-Q,CI	(2)F,F/T,CCD-Q,CI	(3)F,F/T,CCD,CCP-SOM	(4)F,F/T,CCD,CCP-TR	(5)F,F/T,CCD-TR
Inputs	F	-6,51%	0,00%	-40,70%	-8,84%	-7,91%
	CCD	0,00%	-10,09%	0,00%	0,00%	0,00%
	CCP	-45,27%	~	-20,00%	-16,80%	~
	F/T	-8,82%	-15,46%	-7,89%	-26,32%	-32,90%
Outputs	Q	41,47%	38,91%	~	~	~
	CI	11,17%	11,69%	~	~	~
	TR	~	~	~	21,37%	19,36%
	SOM	~	~	21,45%	~	~
Benchmarks	SR4	0,70	~	~	~	~
	SR6	~	~	1,00	~	~
	SR16	~	0,25	~	~	~
	SR 29	~	~	~	~	0,20
	SR32	0,30	0,75	~	~	~
	SR54	~	~	~	0,24	~
	SR59	~	~	~	0,76	0,80
Efficiency		67%	73%	68%	72%	72%

Table 4.3.6-5: Summary of SR 28

Figure 4.3.6-4 depicts the MPI of SR28 for the different versions. The reader may recall that SR28 efficiency development was mainly characterized by a side movement between 0.7 and 0.8, especially in the last eight quarters; before that, the efficiency score was critically low. In the first year SR28 improves the productivity and the efficiency score of SR28 increased. But after that SR28 seems to rest on the laurels. The impression is that SR28 reached a safe position within the sales force and maintains there without using the upward potential this position implies. This assumption can be confirmed by the fact that all MPIs shift relative closely around one during the last eight quarters.

Furthermore, the inclusion and exclusion of CCP has no significant effect on the development of the MPI for SR28. In the last two years the MPI move closely together, regardless which outputs are included into the analysis.

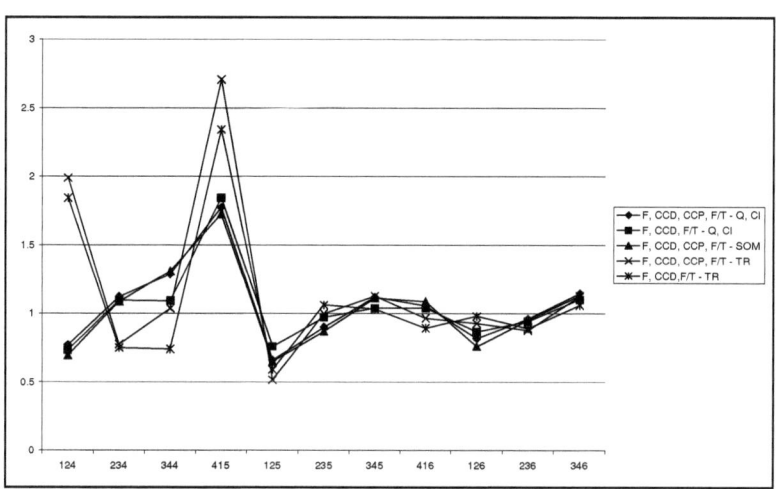

Figure 4.3.6-4: Development of the MPI for the different DEA versions for SR28

Table 4.3.6-6 presents the summary for SR 42. The efficiency scores of SR 42 range between 28% in version (1) and 61% in version (4).

The input F has to be adjusted in versions (5) and (3). The inputs CCD and CCP are chosen optimal in each of the versions by SR42 but the return on CCD and CCP is very low.

An interesting fact is the big difference in the efficiency scores between version (1) and (2) and the other three versions. Obviously the absolute amount of Q is extremely low and that is why it pulls down the efficiency frontier. The data for SR42 in the appendix B confirm this assumption.

The optimal projection of the input F/T differs from the status quo in all versions except in version (3). Therefore the DEA model (3) gives the information that for a focus on market share the input F/T is chosen optimal and in case of other outputs it is not chosen optimal.

Concerning the benchmark partners no dominant benchmark is revealed. In each of the benchmark sets one partner is obviously much better than the others.

SR 42 is very weak in each of the DEA versions. The weakness of SR42 mainly stems from the output side which has to undergo the biggest adjustments for reaching efficiency. These adjustments seem to be unrealistically high and therefore SR42 should leave the company.

SR 42		(1)F,F/T,CCD,CCP-Q,CI	(2)F,F/T,CCD-Q,CI	(3)F,F/T,CCD,CCP-SOM	(4)F,F/T,CCD,CCP-TR	(5)F,F/T,CCD-TR
Inputs	F	0,00%	0,00%	-10,58%	0,00%	-31,90%
	CCD	0,00%	0,00%	0,00%	0,00%	0,00%
	CCP	0,00%	~	0,00%	0,00%	~
	F/T	-15,84%	-18,59%	0,00%	-29,36%	-19,41%
Outputs	Q	435,10%	462,55%	~	~	~
	CI	47,14%	43,63%	~	~	~
	TR	~	~	~	50,84%	44,35%
	SOM	~	~	66,66%	~	~
Benchmarks	SR4	0,19	~	0,05	0,13	~
	SR6	~	~	0,33	~	~
	SR29	~	~	~	~	0,70
	SR32	0,56	0,80	~	~	~
	SR43	0,16	~	0,02	0,09	~
	SR44	~	~	0,61	~	~
	SR54	0,09	0,20	~	0,66	~
	SR59	~	~	~	0,11	0,30
Efficiency		28%	27%	58%	61%	57%

Table 4.3.6-6: Summary of SR 42

For SR42 the inclusion and exclusion of CCP does not have an important impact on the MPI. The high peak at the beginning of 2006 is due to a job rotation. This job rotation was necessary as Figure 4.3.6-5 displays. Compared with the rest of the sample the MPI was weak and often below one. This decreasing total factor productivity resulted in a job rotation. Unfortunately the new sales rep (which was assigned to follow up the job of SR42 by the author) was not much better, despite a very motivated beginning and had to be careful to keep up with the rest of the sample. Similarly to SR4 and 28 the MPI including SOM as output is the lowest which is due to the overall decreasing SOM of the company in the market. This is especially tragic for SR42 because the share of market is already fairly low at the beginning of the time interval.

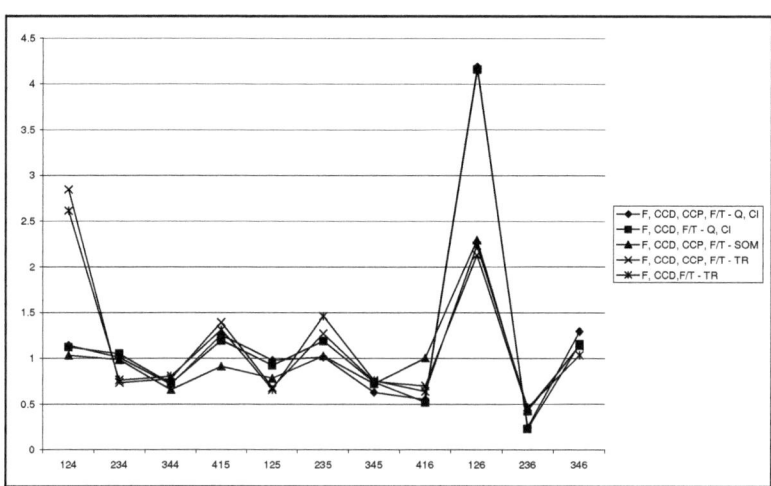

Figure 4.3.6-5: Development of the MPI for the different DEA versions for SR28

Table 4.3.6-7 displays the frequencies of efficient sales reps in the benchmark sets of inefficient sales reps for different DEA versions. In total SR 32 is mentioned 125 times followed by SR6 with 96 times and by SR29 with 56 times. Therefore, from a frequency point of view and considered for all DEA versions, these three sales reps are the most important for evaluating inefficient units. Seven sales reps (6, 23, 29, 43, 48, 54, 59) are efficient in every DEA variant, which makes them the stars of the sales force. The most unimportant sales reps are 15, 30, 57 and 7 who are only mentioned twice or thrice, which indicates that the way their transformation system from inputs to outputs works, differs very much from the "main stream". The highest frequency within a DEA version is achieved by SR32 in version (3). Henceforth SR32 is very important in version (3) as benchmark partner for other sales reps.

Table 4.3.6-8 depicts the cumulated benchmark weights of an efficient sales rep for each DEA version. In total SR 32 weights sum up to an impact factor over all DEA versions of 77.39 followed by SR6 with an impact factor of 50.89 and SR 59 with an impact factor of 29.44.

Sales Reps	(1)F,F/T,CCD,CCP-Q,CI	(2)F,F/T,CCD-Q,CI	(3)F,F/T,CCD,CCP-SOM	(4)F,F/T,CCD,CCP-TR	(5)F,F/T,CCD-TR	Sum
SR4	35	2	4	8	0	49
SR6	5	2	43	34	13	97
SR7	1	1	0	1	0	3
SR15	1	0	1	0	0	2
SR16	2	34	0	0	0	36
SR23	2	4	3	1	3	13
SR27	0	0	0	4	0	4
SR29	2	2	4	14	34	56
SR30	0	0	0	0	2	2
SR32	33	42	0	50	0	125
SR43	11	7	25	5	2	50
SR44	2	2	5	0	0	9
SR46	3	4	3	0	0	10
SR47	1	0	5	1	0	7
SR48	4	5	8	1	1	19
SR54	13	13	1	1	8	36
SR57	1	0	1	1	0	3
SR59	2	4	3	4	33	46
SR62	2	4	2	0	5	13
Sum	120	126	108	125	101	580

Table 4.3.6-7: Frequencies of efficient sales reps in the reference sets of inefficient sales reps in the different DEA versions

Therefore, accounting for the weights instead of the frequency and considered for all DEA versions, these three sales reps are now the most important for evaluating inefficient units. So SR 59 replaced SR 29 in this category compared to the frequency category. The lowest impact is calculated for SR 7, 15, 30 and 57.

For overall sales performance improvement the management is recommended to analyse the stars of the sales force which are indicated by being efficient in every DEA version, by having a high frequency and a high impact value.

Table 4.3.6-9 summarizes the output projections for the whole sample of each DEA version transformed into market share and amount of insulin sold (in MMU). The projected amount of Q sold varies between 511 MMU (+37%) and 437 MMU (+17%) depending on the DEA version applied. The corresponding market share projections vary between 41% (+9 % points) and 35% (+3.2% points).

Sales Reps	(1)F,F/T,CCD,CCP-Q,CI	(2)F,F/T,CCD-Q,CI	(3)F,F/T,CCD,CCP-SOM	(4)F,F/T,CCD,CCP-TR	(5)F,F/T,CCD-TR	Sum
SR4	21,55	1,31	1,60	2,39	0,00	26,85
SR6	2,53	1,01	33,19	7,70	6,47	50,89
SR 7	1,00	1,00	0,00	1,00	0,00	3,00
SR15	1,00	0,00	1,00	0,00	0,00	2,00
SR16	1,09	11,29	0,00	0,00	0,00	12,39
SR23	1,29	2,01	1,36	1,00	1,94	7,60
SR 27	0,00	0,00	0,00	2,06	0,00	2,06
SR29	1,53	1,51	1,79	3,53	15,81	24,16
SR30	0,00	0,00	0,00	0,00	1,42	1,42
SR32	14,04	27,98	0,00	35,37	0,00	77,39
SR43	3,15	2,10	6,86	2,25	1,21	15,58
SR44	1,00	1,22	2,16	0,00	0,00	4,38
SR46	1,82	2,06	1,58	0,00	0,00	5,46
SR47	1,00	0,00	2,37	1,00	0,00	4,37
SR48	1,53	1,73	4,63	1,00	1,59	10,48
SR54	5,03	4,60	1,00	1,00	4,88	16,51
SR57	1,00	0,00	1,00	1,00	0,00	3,00
SR59	1,21	1,41	1,28	1,69	23,85	29,44
SR62	1,23	1,78	1,18	0,00	3,82	8,03
Sum	61,00	61,00	61,00	61,00	61,00	305,00

Table 4.3.6-8: Cumulated weights of the benchmark partners in the reference sets (impact factor)

Therefore the SBM version of DEA identifies a potential market share increase to at least 34,92% by making the inefficient sales reps work as well as the efficient ones in the sample for quarter 4 2006.

SBM DEA Version	Unit	Actual Value	Target Value	Delta	
F,F/T,CCD,CCP-Q,CI	Q	372,70	504,40	35,34%	
	SOM	31,79%	40,29%	8,50	
F,F/T,CCD-Q,CI	Q	373	511	37,01%	
	SOM	32%	41%	9,00	
F,F/T,CCD,CCP-TR	Q	372,70	448,96	20,46%	
	SOM	31,79%	35,86%	4,07	
F,F/T,CCD-TR	Q	372,70	442,36	18,69%	
	SOM	31,79%	35,34%	3,54	
F,F/T,CCD,CCP-SOM	Q	372,70	437,15	17,29%	
	SOM	31,79%	34,92%	3,13	

Table 4.3.6-9: Insulin increases: absolute and in terms of market share

5 Summary and Conclusion

In this thesis, a part of the sales force of a large pharmaceutical company was analysed with regards to efficiency. For this reason Data Envelopment Analysis, which has been applied to various economic and managerial topics in the past (see Taveres 2002), was applied to evaluate the performance of pharmaceutical sales representatives.
DEA has been applied to numerous sales activities (Thomas et al. 1998, Donthu and Yoo 1998, Luo 2003, de Mateo et al. 2006) but it has not been extensively applied to the case of individual salesman performance evaluation. Boles et al. (1995) and Pilling et al. (1999) assess the problem of sales representative evaluation with DEA but they concentrate on a single period using an output orientated CCR model. In addition both of the authors do not account for pharmaceutical sales.
Henceforth a wide range of extensions has been added on top of the existing approaches for sales force evaluation with DEA within this thesis.
At the beginning of the dissertation efficiency concepts were introduced followed by the theoretical basis of non parametric efficiency evaluation. The output orientated CCR, and BCC model were presented next. The calculations of efficiency using the CCR and BCC model were limited to the fourth quarter 2004 and resulted into the conclusion that the CCR model "overestimated" (due to CRS) the optimal output projections which led to unrealistically high target values for the inefficient sales reps. In addition the BCC and CCR model do not include slacks into the resulting efficiency measure and thus, every application of CCR and BCC is forced to divide the sales reps into strong efficient (without slacks) and weak efficient (with slacks) units. This fact reduces the quality of every serious efficiency analysis because for a distinctive ranking the slack values, which are not included into the efficiency measure, have to be weighted externally. Furthermore, concentrating only on output orientated models is questionable, because inputs can be inefficiently high for some sales reps and therefore are worth optimizing.
To overcome these obstacles the non-orientated SBM model with VRS was introduced and applied to the subject. As additional information it was possible to decompose the efficiency score into the contributions of the single input and output dimensions. After the relevant DEA

versions were calculated with the SBM model, inter temporal aspects were highlighted. The needs for an inter-temporal analysis stem mainly from two facts:

1. It is important to trace the efficiency development of sales representatives to reveal trends and tendencies within this development. For example a sales rep who suddenly reaches the efficiency frontier in the current period but which previously had a bad development should not be taken as benchmark for others. The current development may be due to external factors which influenced the efficiency score positively.

2. Another point worth mentioning is the productivity development of the sales force not only on a level regarding all of the sales force but also on an individual level. For this reason the Malmquist Productivity Index was applied to the topic of sales force evaluation. Additional information was discovered by decomposing the MPI in its two components: the catch up process and the frontier shift.

To present the DEA results in a comprehensive way for people who do not have a solid DEA background, the key performance indicator cockpit (or management cockpit) was introduced as tool to evaluate individual sales reps easily. For a global overview on the efficiency characteristics of a sample of units the graphical "efficiency gap" was introduced and discussed.

The theoretical section was followed by a description of the data base which was used for the analysis and where inputs and output are defined. In addition, the currently applied performance evaluation system of the pharmaceutical company is outlined.

After the presentation of the theoretical background, the data base and the current evaluation system, the empirical analysis was conducted.

In the following paragraphs the main questions underlying this thesis will be taken into account with regards to the results of the empirical part.

Of course the first fact to consider was if DEA in general is applicable to the subject of sales forces evaluation in the pharmaceutical industry. During the analysis the topic of sales evaluation with DEA revealed itself to be an interesting alternative to existing benchmarking methods for *every company* with a similar distribution system as soon as both sides of the sales process, the input side and the output side are taken into account. For some firms who only rely on external contractors which are rewarded on commission, only the output side is of interest and therefore a DEA evaluation is not so important.

The most important prerequisite regarding a valid DEA evaluation is to determine inputs and outputs which characterize the sales process and which can be applied to every unit of the sample. This was established in this thesis and as soon as a firm wishes to evaluate individual sales personnel by taking into account multiple inputs and outputs DEA can be recommended.

The data for the inputs and outputs was available quarterly from the first quarter 2004 until to the fourth quarter 2006. Regarding the detailed analysis of the different input and output categories and their contribution to the efficiency score achieved, the focus was directed on to the fourth quarter 2006. To reveal inter-temporal aspects concerning relative efficiency and productivity changes the data range was widened starting in quarter 1 2004 and ending with quarter 4 2006.

In the present analysis four input and four output categories could be evaluated together with the sales managers of the company. The DEA analysis supplied information to identify which sales rep performed efficiently and which one performed inefficiently. Depending on the DEA version applied the different sources of inefficiency could be revealed for the overall sales force and for each and every sales unit.

Due to the great number of individuals, only three sales reps were analysed in detail. The interested reader will find data regarding the SBM DEA version 1 in the appendix B. For the three exemplary sales reps, individual recommendations were given, depending on the DEA version applied. To represent members of each group three sales reps were chosen, one from the group of the efficient 25% (SR4), one from the middle 50% (SR28) and one from the group of the inefficient 25% (SR42).

Summary of the individual sales rep analysis

Next, the attention is turned to Table 5-1 which depicts the (super) efficiency scores for the different DEA models (CCR, BBC and SBM) and versions (1 - 5) of the three sales reps selected.

Version		Rank	DEA Model Efficiency SR4	DEA Model Efficiency SR 28	DEA Model Efficiency SR 42
1 =	F, CCD, CCP, F/T - Q, CI	1	CCR 1 1,98	BCC 2 0,82	BCC 4 0,66
2 =	F, CCD, F/T - Q, CI	2	CCR 4 1,63	BCC 1 0,82	CCR 4 0,65
3 =	F, CCD, CCP, F/T - SOM	3	CCR 3 1,60	BCC 4 0,80	SBM 4 0,61
4 =	F, CCD, CCP, F/T - TR	4	SBM 1 1,29	BCC 3 0,79	BCC 5 0,61
5 =	F, CCD, F/T - TR	5	SBM 3 1,19	CCR 1 0,77	CCR 5 0,60
		6	SBM 4 1,18	CCR 2 0,77	BCC 1 0,60
		7	BCC 2 1,07	CCR 4 0,76	BCC 3 0,60
		8	CCR 2 1,07	BCC 5 0,76	CCR 1 0,60
		9	SBM 2 1,04	CCR 3 0,76	CCR 3 0,60
		10	BCC 1 1,00	CCR 5 0,74	BCC 2 0,59
		11	BCC 4 1,00	SBM 2 0,73	SBM 3 0,58
		12	BCC 3 1,00	SBM 5 0,72	SBM 5 0,57
Table 5-1:Sensitivity of (super) efficiency scores to changes in the DEA models and versions		13	BCC 5 0,87	SBM 4 0,72	CCR 2 0,57
		14	CCR 5 0,84	SBM 3 0,68	SBM 1 0,28
		15	SBM 5 0,83	SBM 1 0,67	SBM 2 0,27

It is obvious that the results of the efficiency analysis depend very much on the DEA version chosen.

For example SR4 attained the worst efficiency score for all models with the version 5 input and output mix. This must be due to the fact that both the exclusion of CCP and the inclusion of TR have a negative influence on the efficiency score. The versions 1, 3 and 4 are ranked the highest for the CCR and SBM model (rank 1 - 6). These versions have in common that they include CCP on the input side. In the BCC model the versions 1, 3 and 4 are ranked 10 to 12. Hence, for SR4 the output orientated BCC model seems to be unfavourable. However in the BCC versions 1, 3 and 4 SR4 is still efficient and exactly hits the efficiency frontier. The exclusion of SR4 does not change the frontier and therefore the efficiency score must be one. A look at the outcomes of SR28 reveals that the SBM model is the strictest efficiency measure. Regarding the CCR and BCC model the versions 2 and 1 result in the highest scores. Interestingly this fact is different for the SBM model because the highest score is attained by version 2 and the lowest by version one. This is due to the fact that the SBM model is input and output orientated. Therefore there is only one conclusion: SR28 uses *relatively* high amounts of the input CCP. This is not so important for the output orientated models and therefore version 1 and 2 are the best in the CCR and BCC model. Considering the SBM model this fact differs. The input side is optimized as well and therefore a high CCP value influences the efficiency score negatively. That is why version 2 (excluding CCP) is the best of the SBM models and version 1 (including CCP) is the worst.

SR42 has the best results for the version 4 models. Therefore the output "target realization" in combination with the input CCP makes SR42 achieve the best efficiency score. The output combination of Q and CI decreases the efficiency. The worst efficiency scores are attained when Q and CI are included as outputs and CCP is excluded from the evaluation. This combination always achieves the worst results in one of the three DEA models.

In case the efficiency sore is smaller than one, the SBM model is always the strictest benchmarking method.

These findings are confirmed in detail by the key performance indicator cockpits in the corresponding chapters of the empirical part of the thesis.

This kind of summarized sensitivity analysis could be applied to all of the 61 sales reps in the sample. In contrast to the virtual weights which show the leverage effect of a dimension on efficiency, the inclusion or exclusion of dimensions directly show an impact on efficiency and hence directly reveal the relative strength or weakness of a sales rep within that dimension in comparison to the rest of the sample.

Table 5-1 casts light on the detail that the efficiency scores reveal a high sensitivity to changes in the DEA settings. Consequently it is crucial to find an adequate model and version for evaluating the sales force efficiency.

However, if a suitable model is found, the sales management is able to identify which dimension includes the greatest inefficiency for every inefficient sales rep and therefore can recommend where to start with efficiency improvements. As an example the implications of a step wise improvement in the inefficient dimensions for SR 28 is displayed in Figure 5-1 below. On the vertical axes the efficiency is displayed and on the horizontal axes the different improvement steps. In a first step the inefficiency in the input F is deleted. As a consequence the efficiency score rises by 1.8% points. In a next step the inefficiency of the input CCP is deleted which leads to an increased score by 3.5% points.

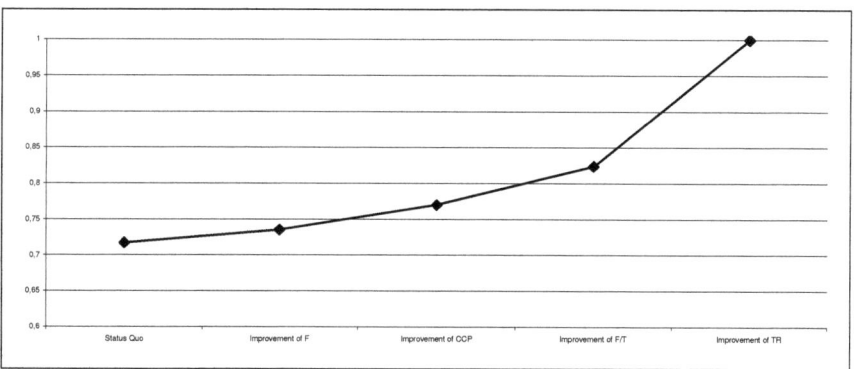

Figure 5-1: Increase in efficiency for SR28 by deleting the inefficiencies in the specific dimensions (Model: SBM; Version: F, CCD, CCP, F/T-TR)

The improvement in the factor F/T implies a rise in the efficiency score by 5.4% points. Finally the improvement of TR results in an increase of 17.6% points.

Therefore the sales management could recommend that SR28 should start improving the output TR first, because this output dimension is responsible for the greatest decrease in efficiency. This kind of recommendation can be applied to each and every sales rep and will clearly enhance the entire sales force performance on both, the input and output side, if the sales reps are able to implement the advices.

DEA Model selection

Regarding the already described possibility of overestimated optimal projections in the CCR models, the focus on outputs only and the problems stemming from distinguishing weak from strong efficient units (BCC and CCR), it is straightforward to concentrate on the non orientated SBM model with VRS. Due to VRS the optimal projections can not be overestimated. Because of the inclusion of slacks no distinction between weak and strong efficient units is necessary and the non orientation guarantees an optimization in both directions[23].

---

[23] For a detailed discussion on the model characteristics the interested reader is referred to chapter two.

Once a DEA model is identified the input and output structure has to be chosen. In this thesis five different versions were tested using three different models. The SBM model has been identified as the most suitable.

Selection of an appropriate DEA version

The next problem to solve is which input and output mix is to be chosen? Beside others Pedraja-Chaparro (1999) and Wilson (1995) point out that the user of DEA has little available guidance on the model quality. Methods like misspecification tests or goodness of fit statistics developed for parametric statistical methods are not offered by the DEA technique. Yet, if a DEA model is used for managerial reasons, the quality of the model is of crucial importance. Attributing the fact that no DEA quality testing instruments are available the modelling context is of crucial importance in judging whether a DEA model is likely to be satisfactory.

Considering the fact that for specific reasons the SBM model is more suitable the choice is between five different input and output mixes. For identifying the best model the following two approaches are suggested:

1. Economic meaningfulness

    The five output mixes all are economically sensible but lead to different efficiency results. Hence the management must carefully decide where to put the focus on. If the focus on the output side is put upon absolute sales of insulin, the output Q should be taken into account. If the output Q shall be adjusted for different territory potential the output CI (Competition Index) can be added. If the spotlight is on market share the output SOM (Share of Market) should be chosen and if the output TR (Target Realization) is of concern it should be added to the analysis. The same holds for the input side. The input combination which reflects the characteristics of the sales process best should be chosen.

2. Variation of inputs and outputs

    By varying the inputs and outputs the sensibility of the results to data variations can be revealed. In case a variation of inputs leads to limited changes within the results only little additional information was gained by this variation. For the present analysis Table 5-2 displays basic characteristics for the five SBM versions. If the sales management wishes a version with a high discriminatory power to clearly distinguish between sales reps regarding efficiency it should seek out for a DEA version with a low average efficiency and a high standard deviation. In that case version 1 should be selected. In case the sales management wants to put pressure for improvement on a wider range of sales reps it should rather apply models with a small number of efficient units like version 5.

Model: NO-SBM-V	(1) F, CCD, CCP, F/T - Q,CI	(2) F, CCD, F/T - Q,CI	(3) F, CCD, CCP, F/T - SOM	(4) F, CCD, CCP, F/T - TR	(5) F, CCD, F/T – TR
Ø Efficiency	0.735	0.757	0.756	0.763	0.763
Standard Deviation	0.198	0.177	0.166	0.152	0.138
Number of Efficient Units	13	11	10	8	7

Table 5-2: Characteristic determinants of the different DEA versions

The previous paragraphs evaluated model selection approaches regarding a single period; in this case the fourth quarter 2006. Taking into account points 1 and 2 the selection of an adequate DEA model very much depends on the preferences of the user and therefore no general rule can be stated.

Conclusion on the input and output dimensions chosen

Table 5-3 summarizes the results of the Mann Whitney U Tests applied to the SBM versions to detect the main drivers of the average efficiency scores of the efficient 25%, the middle 50% and the inefficient 25% of the sales reps.

Table 5-3 should be interpreted the following way: The higher the efficiency score for a unit is the higher the virtual weight of the specific dimensions of that unit should be. Therefore, if the virtual weight of a dimension seems to be randomly scattered, no matter which efficiency score a unit attained, the specific dimension does not seem to be relevant for a high efficiency score. In other words, all of the groups use this input with a similar intensity and therefore the overall optimization potential is not that big. But if the highest virtual weights for a dimension are detected in the group of the efficient 25% of the sales reps, this finding indicates that the efficient group uses that factor more intensely than the other groups do. Henceforth this factor can be viewed as one reason for the higher efficiency score of the top group.

If a significant difference was detected between two efficiency groups regarding the average virtual weights in a dimension, the group with the higher mean rank worked more efficiently than the others in that dimension. All SBM DEA versions were analysed to find these significant differences between the three efficiency groups according to the U-Test. In case a significant difference at the level $p \leq 5\%$ between two groups regarding an input or output dimension was detected, a "1" was assigned to this specific dimensions in Table 5-3 otherwise "0" standing for no significance. These values (1 or 0) are displayed from the second column onwards in Table 5-3. For example the output CI in version 2 has been assigned a 1 for each of the three group comparisons. The 1 indicates that significant differences regarding the virtual prices of the output dimension CI exist, in the sense that the mean rank for the efficient 25% is higher than for the middle 50% and the inefficient 25%. In addition the average virtual weight of the output CI of the middle 50% is significantly different (higher) than the weight of the inefficient 25%. Hence the attendance of a sales rep to the efficient 25% means that he or she was on average better in producing the output CI than members of the other two groups. Thus, if a "1" is assigned to a comparison there is a significantly positive connection between average efficiency scores and average virtual weights.

DEA Version	Group Comparison	F	CCD	CCP	F/T	Q	CI	TR	SOM
1	A vs B	1	0	1	1	1	1	~	~
	A vs C	1	0	1	1	1	1	~	~
	B vs C	0	0	0	0	0	1	~	~
2	A vs B	0	0	~	1	1	1	~	~
	A vs C	0	0	~	1	1	1	~	~
	B vs C	0	0	~	0	0	1	~	~
3	A vs B	0	0	1	1	~	~	~	1
	A vs C	0	1	1	1	~	~	~	1
	B vs C	0	0	0	0	~	~	~	0
4	A vs B	0	1	1	1	~	~	1	~
	A vs C	0	1	1	1	~	~	1	~
	B vs C	0	0	0	0	~	~	0	~
5	A vs B	0	1	~	1	~	~	1	~
	A vs C	0	1	~	1	~	~	1	~
	B vs C	0	0	~	0	~	~	0	~

Table 5-3: Characteristic differences between groups regarding efficiency for the SBM model, q4 2006 (efficient 25% = A; middle 50% = B; inefficient 25%= C)

Except for version 1 the average virtual weights of the input F do not differ significantly between the efficiency groups. This finding leads to the assumption that no matter which efficiency group sales reps are in, they use the input F in a similar intensity and therefore there is almost no connection between average efficiency scores and average virtual weights of F.

In versions one, two and three no significant differences regarding the input CCD are detected which leads to a similar conclusion as for the input F. However, if TR is introduced as output the efficient 25% differ significantly from the other groups. Thus, with TR as output the intensity of the use of the input CCD seems to be significantly different between the quartiles.

The virtual weight of the input CCP differs significantly between the top group and the two other groups in every application and hence high virtual weights of CCP indicate high average efficiency scores. This leads to the conclusion that in each version when CCP is included, the efficient 25% make use of it in the best way. This finding indicates a lot of improvement potential by cutting down CCP in the middle and inefficient group.

The input F/T is included in every version and always reveals itself to have a high discriminatory power regarding the virtual weights between the quartiles. The results show that the top group always has the higher virtual prices as the other two efficiency groups and therefore the mean rank regarding the virtual weights is significantly different for each DEA version. This indicates that an optimal F/T value lies beneath the proposed target value of 0.8 which is recommended by the sales management.

The characteristics concerning the virtual weight of output Q lead to a similar conclusion. When it is included the mean rank of the group regarding Q indicates a high discriminatory power between the top group and the other groups and hence the efficient 25% are therefore better in producing Q than the rest of the sample.

The same conclusion holds for the outputs TR and SOM.

The output CI in version 1 and 2 is special in the sense that the average virtual weights are discriminated significantly between all of the groups and not only between the top group and the two other groups. This finding highlights the fact that a sales rep faces competition in average better the higher the efficiency score is.

For a sales manager the conclusion regarding the inputs and outputs would have the following implication:

> Attributing the inputs CCP and F/T, the sales manager should try to examine why the efficient group is so much better in the use of these inputs in all of the versions.
> Regarding the input F the question arises why the sales force cannot be differentiated regarding efficiency by this output.
> Concerning the input CCD, the reason for the rising discriminating power, when the input TR is included, is worth examining.
> The question arising on the output side is if the efficient sales reps are better in selling due to the quality of their inputs (which is indicated for each sales rep and for each dimensions through the virtual weight for that dimension) or maybe because of favourable external conditions in the sense that the doctors contacted for some reason buy more than in other regions.

It is worth mentioning that the outcomes of the input CCD (it does not differ between the groups for some DEA versions) do not mean that it is not important for the production of outputs but it means that it has a similar importance for all of the groups and therefore does not have a high discriminating power regarding efficiency similar to the input F.

In this thesis there is no answer to the question *why* a sales rep is inefficient in a category, but the question in *which* category a sales rep is inefficient in relation to the best performers is answered. The answer to the why only can be give by additional qualitative research effort which is not part of this thesis.

The MPI and sales force evaluation

In this thesis the MPI was used to examine the changes in total factor productivity of sales reps over a certain space in time. The non orientated, slack based Super-MPI with VRS was applied to overcome major shortcomings of current empirical DEA studies, which were presented in chapter 2.
The MPI revealed itself to be a useful instrument in the analysis of a sales force. For each sales rep the TFP was examined for different DEA versions. Through the variation of inputs

and outputs the effects on TFP could be detected. This was one method used to detect the influence of different variables on the development of the MPI of individual sales reps. Strong performing sales reps are characterized by an MPI which remains above one. Such sales reps are increasing productivity from period to period which can either reflects in an increasing efficiency score from period to period or by the fact that such a sales rep "drags out" the efficiency frontier. This would encourage the other sales rep to close up so that they do not decrease in their efficiency scores.

Weak performing sales reps are characterized by an MPI below one. This is reflected in decreasing efficiency scores and could finally result in the sales rep leaving the company.

An interesting question, as to how the static efficiency score and the inter-temporal MPI could be combined into a measure for evaluating a sales rep, remains to be solved. It is important for a sales rep not only to be evaluated on the bases of a single period but also on the bases of former performance development. Therefore a combined measure of both performance indicators MPI and efficiency score of the last period like: "Final score of SR = 0.3xMPI+0.7xEfficiencyScore" could be introduced. But of course, the weights for such a procedure would be chosen subjective again. Another approach could be to pay a bonus for a good development of the MPI and to base the main evaluation of sales reps solely on the efficiency score.

For the reasons mentioned above the MPI adds an additional and useful tool to sales force evaluation and, hence, can be used in practical applications.

The DEA method in comparison to the current evaluation method

The current evaluation methods had several shortcomings presented in chapter 3.2. In this section these shortcomings will be discussed in the light of DEA.

For the evaluation of the sales rep the pharmaceutical company divided the input and output dimension into intervals. These intervals where created subjectively. The importance in setting these intervals is to set them in such a way that they are not impossible to reach and do not discourage the sales force. Depending on the interval the value of a dimension for a sales rep lay in the sales rep reaching a certain amount of points. These points were again set subjectively in the best practice manner. Each of the dimensions was assigned a different weight. From the view of the sales management these weights reflected the importance of a dimension for the sales process. Further more these weights were chosen for each dimension and not for each sales rep. The overall score of a sales rep was calculated by multiplying the weights of each dimension with the points a sales rep achieved within that dimension. For the final conclusion of a sales rep, all of the weighted points where summed up in a final score, which ranged between 0 and 5.

The intervals, the points and the weights are created subjectively and are based on best practice experiences. Therefore, it remains uncertain if the achieved score of a sales rep reflects reality in comparison with the rest of the sample or if the achieved score is heavily influenced by misjudgements and inefficiencies underlying the set up of intervals, points and weights.

DEA for instance, does not rely on intervals and points which are not necessary in the DEA sales force evaluation process. DEA calculates individual weights as part of an objective optimization program which *maximise* the efficiency score of an individual with respect to the rest of the sample for every sales rep. The weights DEA assigns to sales reps for the dimensions cannot be better chosen by the management, only could be found by chance. Therefore, DEA provides a holistic tool, in which misjudgements, due to subjectively chosen indicators, are avoided!

Furthermore, the focus lay on effectiveness rather than on efficiency (see Figure 2.2.1-1). That means that the sales rep had to reach certain input targets no matter if these targets where necessary or not, for achieving the output results. The intuition behind this evaluation is that high inputs guarantee high outputs. This view upon the sales process can lead to a misallocation of resources. Sales reps can be encouraged to increase the input quantity as high as possible in order to compensate for bad sales results, because the points for the sales rep evaluation on the input side increase with increasing inputs, which in turn improves the overall evaluation score. This behaviour will lead to an additional decrease on the marginal return of an input unit and therefore, to a loss of sales quality. Therefore, a concentration on effectiveness leads to problematical incentives. If the focus is rather on efficiency though this guarantees high quality of inputs and, as the numerous optimal projections revealed, improves sales success. This improvement amounts to at least 3% additional market share (see chapter 4.3.6).

Besides the advantages stated above, DEA can account for additional positive points. The current evaluation method cannot be used to forecasting and quantifying the losses due to inefficient operation. In contrast, DEA calculates optimal target values for each sales rep by comparing fairly with the "best in class" counterparts and thus quantifies the "opportunity costs of inefficiency". These optimal projections cannot be quantified by the method currently used.

DEA analyses the sales force from an efficiency point of view and identifies those sales rep with the best marginal return on effort, indicating high salesmanship skills. This is not achieved by the method currently used.

Furthermore, DEA identifies benchmark partners for the inefficient sales reps, who can be viewed as mentors for increasing the sales performance of inefficient sales reps.

In case a sales rep is inefficient, this inefficiency can be decomposed into the different components. The more a dimension of a sales rep contributes to the inefficiency, the more improvement potential this dimension implies.

Furthermore, DEA can be used for inter-temporal sales force analysis as well. This goes beyond the static approach of the current evaluation system. With the help of the MPI, changing productivity of the whole sample and of individual sales reps can be traced as chapter 4.3 presented. This feature is helpful for controlling the effects of past sales management decisions on the whole sample, and for identifying the source of the productivity increase of a sales rep: Is the productivity increase due to positive frontier shift or due to more efficient operations of the sales rep?

Disadvantages of DEA

The author suggests that the DEA benchmarking method gives a better overview over the sales force performance than the method currently used, because it does not just concentrate on the output or the input side, but on both sides simultaneously. In addition, the advantages stated above constitute strong arguments pro DEA.

However, every method has its shortcomings. The weakness with the DEA method is that it is sensitive to outliers. As a consequence two sales reps had to be excluded from the sample because their data set revealed irregular data due to the fact that these two sales reps only worked one month of quarter 4 2006 and therefore had to low inputs. A possible result could be that a sales rep, which has very low inputs (due to illness etc.), could turn out to be the most efficient one, because the relationship between inputs and output is the best. Therefore, it is important to have a good overview of the sales force within a sample, in order to adjust for irregularities.

For high quality DEA results it is important to have a sample size which exceeds the number of the sum of inputs and outputs times three (see Tone 2007). Therefore, a "critical" size of the sample is needed with regards to the number of dimensions and only if this critical size is it is sensible to apply a DEA.

In addition, the fact that no measure of quality exists, like in parametrical methods imposes challenges in finding the best DEA setting. From the view of the author the subjectivity, which does not occur within the DEA process, is replaced at an earlier stage of the DEA analysis, being be found in the choice of inputs and outputs. Due to the fact that there does not exist a measure of quality (like the R^2 in regression methods) which clearly indicates which DEA version is the best, the choice of inputs and outputs is one of the most important points within a DEA application.

Summing up

To conclude, DEA could perhaps be a powerful tool in control for relative efficiency and, using the MPI, productivity developments within the sales force.

Current situation:	vs.	Situation using DEA:
▪ Several different benchmarks to evaluate sales representatives		▪ One single Benchmark incorporating all questions of concern
▪ Every single benchmark only highlights one specific view upon a topic		▪ DEA-benchmarking considers multiple inputs and outputs providing a complete picture of the performance of each sales unit in comparison to all the others
▪ Which benchmark is the most important?		▪ Through unbiased weights calculated endogenously DEA identifies those inputs/outputs which have the biggest impact on efficiency
▪ Deficits in evaluating a single benchmark incorporating all relevant inputs and outputs in the right manner.		▪ DEA: Providing a holistic, objective benchmarking tool

In addition, DEA is the first instrument to ***quantify the opportunity costs of inefficiency*** or, in other words, shows ***upwards sales potential*** triggered by increasing sales operations efficiency. Therefore, DEA helps to use existing capacity more intensively!

Furthermore, the DEA method can be extended and modified through additional quantitative (e.g. market size) or qualitative measures (e.g. salesmanship, IQ of SR, customer satisfaction).

DEA is not only powerful on the level of individual sales reps, but also on every other level of the sales force for which equal inputs and outputs can be identified. Perhaps DEA can be applied to a totally different field of operations as well. Examples could be the evaluation of research departments, production lines, country affiliates or even international comparisons between insulin sales forces etc.

6 References

Andersen, P and Petersen, N.C., (1993), "A procedure for ranking efficient units in data envelopment analysis," *Management Science* 39, 1261-1264.

Avila, Ramon A., Edward F. Fern and O. Karl Mann (1988),"Unravelling Criteria for Assessing the Performance of Salespeople," *Journal of Personal Selling and Sales Management*, 8 (May), 45-54

Bagozzi, Richard P. (1978), "Sales Force Performance and Satisfaction as a Function of Individual Difference, Interpersonal, and Situational Factors", *Journal of Personal Selling and Sales Management*, 8 (May), 45 -54

Banker R. D.; Charnes A.; Cooper W. W. (1984), "Some Models for Estimating Technical and Scale Inefficiencies in Data Envelopment Analysis", *Management Science*, Vol. 30, No. 9, pp. 1078-1092

Banker, Rajiv A., Morey, Richard C. (1985), "Efficiency Analysis for exogenously fixed inputs and outputs", *Operations Research*, 34 (July – August), 4

Boles, James S., Naveen Donthu and Ritu Lohtia (1995), "Salesperson Evaluation Using Relative Performance Efficiency: The Application of Data Envelopment Analysis," *Journal of Personal Selling and Sales Management*, 15, 3, 38-49.

Chen, Yao (2003), A non-radial Malmquist productivity index with an illustrative application to Chinese major industries Int. *J. Production Economics* 83 (2003) 27–35

Cooper, William W., Seiford, Lawrence M., Tone, Kaoru (2006) "Introduction to Data Envelopment Analysis and Its Uses: With DEA-Solver Software and References", *Springer*

Churchill, Gilbert A. Jr., Neil M. Ford, Steve W. Hartley and Orvill C. Walker, Jr. (1985), "The Determinants of Salespersons Performance: A Meta Analysis", *Journal of Marketing Research*, V22 (May), 103-118

Churchill, Gilbert A. Jr. and Orvill C. Walker, Jr., (1990), *Sales Force Management*, 3ed, Homewood, IL: Irwin

Charnes, A.C., W.W. Cooper and E. Rhodes (1978), "Measuring the Efficiency of Decision Making Units," *European Journal of Operational Research*, 3, 6, 429-444.

Charnes, A.C., C.T. Clark, W.W. Cooper and B. Golany (1985b), "A Developmental Study of Data Envelopment Analysis in Measuring the Efficiency of Maintenance Units in the U.S. Air Forces," *Annals of Operations Research*, 2, 95-112.

Chonko, Lawrence B., Terry N. Loe, James A. Roberts and John F. Tanner (2000), "Sales Performance: Timing of Measurement and Type of Measurement Make a Difference," *Journal of Personal Selling and Sales Management*, 10, 1, 23-36.

Cocanaugher, A. Benton and John M. Ivanchevich (1978), "BARS Performance Rating for Sales Force Personnel", *Journal of Marketing*, 42 (July), 87-95

Cooper W., Seiford, L.M. and Tone K. (2006), "*Data Envelopment Analysis: A Comprehensive Text with Models, Applications, References and DEA-Solver Software*", Second Edition, Springer

Cravens, David W., Raymond W. Laforge, Gregory M. Pickett and Clifford E. Young (1993), "Incorporating a Quality Improvement Perspective into Measures of Salesperson Performance", *Journal of Personal Selling and Sales Management*, 13 (Winter), 1-14

De Mateo, Filadelfo, Coelli, Tim and O'Donnell, Chris (2006),"Optimal paths and costs of adjustment in dynamic DEA models: with application to chilean department stores", *Annals of Operations Research,* 145, 211-227

Donthu, Naveen and Bonghee Yoo (1998), "Retail Productivity Assessment: Using Data Envelopment Analysis," *Journal of Retailing*, 74, 1, 89-117.

Eichel, E. and H. E. Bender (1984), *Performance Appraisal: A Study of Current Techniques*, New York: American Management Association

Eviews 4.1 Student Version (2004), Quantitative Microsoftware LLC, Irvine, USA

Farrell, M. J. (1957). "The Measurement of Productive Efficiency", *Journal of the Royal Statistical Scociety*, 120:253–81.

Färe, R., S. Grosskopf, B. Lindgren und P. Roos (1994), "Productivity Developments in Swedish Hospitals: A Malmquist Output Index Approach", In A. Charnes, W. W.
Cooper, A. Y. Lewin und L. M. Seiford, Hg., *Data Envelopment Analysis. Theory, Methodology and Applications*, 253–72. Boston, Dordrecht, London: Kluwer Academic Publishers.

Hastings, Bill, Julia Kiely, and Trevor Watkins (1988),"Sales Force Motivation Using Travel Incentives: Some Empirical Evidence", *Journal of Personal Selling and Sales Management*, 8 (August), 43-51

Hollander, Myles and Wolfe, Douglas A, Non parametrical Statistical Methods – 2nd Edition, John Whiley & Sons, Canada

Horsky, Dan and Paul Nelson (1996), "Evaluation of Salesforce Size and Productivity Through Efficient Frontier Benchmarking," *Marketing Science*, 15, 4, 301-321.

Hoy, Michael, Livernois, John and McKenna, Chris (2002), Mathematics for Economics – 2nd Edition, *The MIT Press*

Kohli, Ajay K. (1989), "Effects of Supervisory Behavior: The Role of Individual Differences among Salespeople", *Journal of Marketing*, 53 (October), 40-50

Koopmans, T. C. (1951). An Analysis of Production as an Efficient Combination of Activities. In T. C. Koopmans, Hg., *Activity Analysis of Production and Allocation*, 33–97. New York, London: John-Wiley and Sons, Inc.

Lawrence M. Lamont and William J. Lundstrom, "Identifying Successful Industrial Salesmen by Personality and Personal Characteristics", *Journal of Marketing Research* Vol. XIV (November 1977), 517 - 29

Lucas, Henry C., Jr., Charles B. Weinberg, and Kenneth W. Clowes (1975), „Sales Response as a Function of Territorial Potential and Sales Representative Workload", *Journal of Marketing Research*, 12 (August), 298-305

Luo, Xueming (2003), "Evaluating the Profitability and Marketability Efficiency of Large Banks: An Application of Data Envelopment Analysis," *Journal of Business Research*, 56, 627-635

Meyer, J.-A. (1999), „Visualisierung von Informationen", *Gabler*, Wiesbaden

Pareto, V. (1897). Cours d'´economie politique, Band 2. Lausanne.

Pedraja-Chaparro, F., Salinas-JimeÂnez J., and Smith P. (1999), "On the quality of the data envelopment analysis model", *Journal of the Operational Research Society 50*, 636-644

Pilling, Bruce K., Naveen Donthu and Henson, Steve (1999), "Accounting for the Impact ofTerritory Characteristics on Sales Performance: Relative Efficiency as a Measure of Salesperson Performance," *Journal of Personal Selling and Sales Management*, 19, 2, 35-45.

Ray, Subhash C (2004): "*Data Envelopment Analysis: Theory and Techniques for Economics and Operations Research*", Cambridge University Press

Schumacher, Reiß (2006): „Innovative Pharmaindustrie als Chance für den Wirtschaftsstandort Deutschland", *German Association of research-based pharmaceutical companies, Frauenhofinstitut*, p. 54

Thanasoullis, Emmanuell (2001), "Introduction to the Theory and Application of Data Envelopment Analysis - A Foundation Text with Integrated Software", *Springer*, 1 edition

Tavares, Gabriel (2002), "A Bibliography of Data Envelopment Analysis", *Rutcor Research Report*, 01-02

Tone, Kaoru (2001), "A slacks-based measure of efficiency in data envelopment analysis", *European Journal of Operational Research,* 130, 498-509.

Tone, Kaoru (2002), "A slacks-based measure of super-efficiency in data envelopment analysis", *European Journal of Operational Research,* 143, 32-41.

Thomas, Rhonda R., Richard S. Barr, William L. Cron and John W. Slocum, Jr. (1998), "A Process for Evaluating Retail Store Efficiency: A Restricted DEA Approach," *International Journal of Research in Marketing*, 15, 5, 487-503.

Sager, Jeffrey and Varadarajan, Rajan (1990), "The Fine Art of Performance Appraisal: The Art of Overkill", *Akron Business and Economic Review*, 21 (Spring), 38-50

VassarStats, Online Software, (2007), http://faculty.vassar.edu/lowry/utest.html, Vassar College, New York, USA

Weeks, William A. and Lyon R. Kahle (1990),"Salespeople's Time Use and Performance", *Journal of Personal Selling and Sales Management*, 10 (February), 29-37

Wilson, Paul W. (1995), "Detecting influential observation in data envelopment analysis", *Journal of Productivity Analysis* 6, (1): 27-45

Zhu, Joe, (2002), "*Quantitative Models for Performance Evaluation and Benchmarking: Data Envelopment Analysis with Spreadsheets and DEA Excel Solver*", Springer Netherland

7 Appendix

7.1 Appendix A

DMU	Data			CCR	SBM	Super-SBM
	x1	x2	y			
A	4	3	1	0.8571	0.8333	
B	7	3	1	0.6316	0.6191	
C	8	1	1	1	1	1.125
D	4	2	1	1	1	1.25
E	2	4	1	1	1	1.5
F	10	1	1	1	0.9	

Table 7.2-1: Super Efficiency Datasheet – Input orientated with CCR and SBM results

This example consists of six DMUs with two inputs x_1 and x_2 and one output y which is standardized to 1. The input orientated CCR score is listed in the column CCR in the table. The CCR model identifies the DMU F as weak efficient (1), because it has a slack in x_1 against C. The SBM input orientated CRS model uncovers this slack and assigns a score of 0.9 to F. Hence, C, D and E are identified as truly efficient. Figure 7.2-1 displays the production possibility set P formed by the six DMUs along with the efficient frontiers.

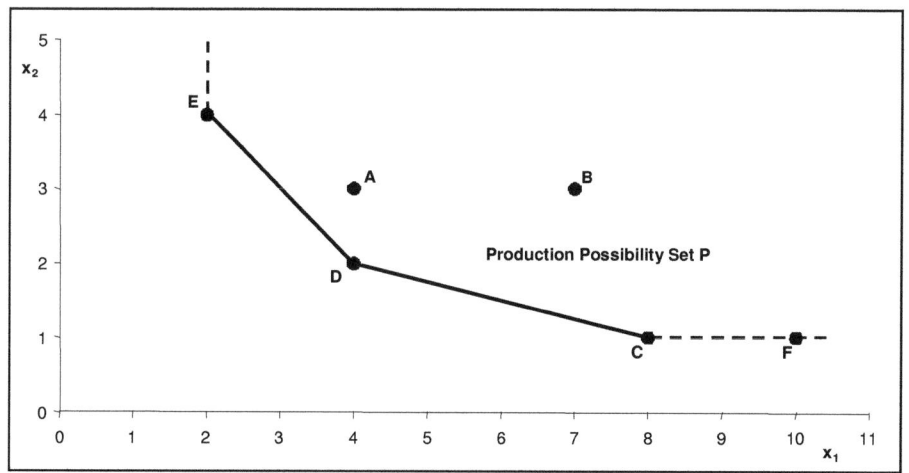

Figure 7.2-1: Production possibility set P and frontiers

Figure 7.2-2 depicts the production possibility set P' formed by excluding D from the DMU set. Let (x_1', x_2', y') be a point in P'. With $x_1'=4,4$, $x_2'=2,8$ and $y'=y=1$.

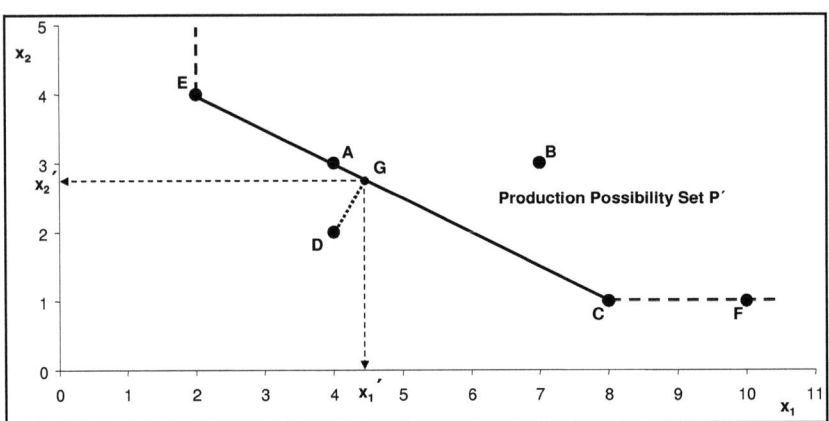

Figure 7.2-2: Production possibility set P' and frontiers

Corresponding to chapter 2.4.4 the distance in the input space between D and G (x_1', x_2', y') is defined as $\left(\dfrac{x_1'}{x_{1D}} + \dfrac{x_2'}{x_{2D}}\right)\dfrac{1}{2}$. Where two denotes the number of inputs.

In accordance with 2.4.4 the distance between D and P' is defined as the optimal value of the following program:

$$\min\left(\frac{x_1'}{x_{1D}} + \frac{x_2'}{x_{2D}}\right)\frac{1}{2}$$

s.t. (B1)

$$\begin{pmatrix} x_1' \\ x_2' \end{pmatrix} \geq \lambda_A \begin{pmatrix} x_{1A} \\ x_{2A} \end{pmatrix} + \lambda_C \begin{pmatrix} x_{1C} \\ x_{2C} \end{pmatrix}$$

$$x_1' \geq x_{1D}$$

$$x_2' \geq x_{2D}$$

$$y' = y_D$$

$$(x_1', x_2', y') \in P'$$

The optimal solution is denoted by the point G in Figure B-2 with $x_1'=4,4$, $x_2'=2,8$, and $y'=1$. Solving the program (B1) the distance is $(4,4/4+2,8/2)/2=1.25$. Similarly, the distances of the other DMU can be measured, i.e., the super-efficiency, of C and D as shown in Table B1. In this example, the ranking of DMUs is E, D, C, F, A, and B in this order.

7.2 Appendix B

DMU	(I)F	(I)CCD	(I)CCP	(I)F/T	(O)Q	(O)SOM/CI	(O)TR
SR1	62%	200	120	83%	6,785505543	34,99%	96,11%
SR2	84%	273	84	100%	6,200005511	27,91%	87,69%
SR3	93%	200	140	68%	5,778505378	27,47%	75,54%
SR4	75%	240	40	72%	9,487008958	35,94%	105,41%
SR5	77%	200	80	85%	4,250004155	22,32%	75,76%
SR6	51%	228	76	70%	6,482005901	38,93%	108,14%
SR7	65%	240	100	60%	6,714506404	33,89%	101,73%
SR8	90%	240	160	83%	5,122004608	28,68%	75,32%
SR9	68%	240	140	71%	8,262007773	37,06%	104,58%
SR10	92%	270	90	92%	8,093507406	32,71%	103,89%
SR11	91%	180	100	100%	7,655006816	24,99%	85,25%
SR12	84%	190	76	85%	7,793007353	35,44%	105,41%
SR13	87%	228	133	74%	4,561504022	25,36%	74,86%
SR14	67%	220	80	84%	5,25200477	31,55%	91,34%
SR15	90%	228	95	80%	4,247003738	41,20%	108,93%
SR16	65%	220	100	68%	7,727007101	38,46%	100,48%
SR17	76%	209	114	81%	5,536004893	28,10%	112,17%
SR18	72%	220	80	92%	6,150005169	27,19%	85,42%
SR19	65%	190	95	100%	5,681005295	26,95%	88,35%
SR20	85%	260	160	94%	4,817004587	40,80%	116,63%
SR21	93%	210	90	82%	5,955505576	28,77%	91,13%
SR22	95%	228	76	86%	7,596506779	33,67%	100,92%
SR23	88%	140	120	73%	6,165505276	31,19%	89,23%
SR24	75%	240	100	91%	7,258506854	31,49%	105,22%
SR26	93%	266	152	85%	7,155006822	31,42%	110,93%
SR27	64%	162	108	79%	5,163504568	26,59%	85,07%
SR28	86%	228	95	76%	6,831006513	32,05%	96,21%
SR29	44%	180	90	79%	4,946504445	28,61%	98,93%
SR30	97%	231	147	66%	6,653006285	39,77%	131,74%
SR32	93%	200	80	63%	10,07650883	34,91%	104,96%
SR33	62%	200	100	92%	4,84150434	26,53%	80,69%
SR34	86%	220	100	89%	3,561503245	37,18%	92,51%
SR35	72%	200	100	80%	4,030503491	29,59%	83,36%
SR36	95%	200	120	74%	7,432006642	34,56%	102,15%
SR37	89%	220	80	82%	4,06250347	21,32%	60,92%
SR38	79%	200	60	92%	5,774005301	31,51%	97,21%
SR39	86%	280	160	84%	7,019506467	35,34%	97,29%
SR40	92%	234	72	87%	6,997506636	34,33%	100,49%
SR41	86%	280	80	81%	6,123005829	32,45%	96,70%
SR42	84%	198	72	85%	1,687001572	23,85%	72,67%
SR43	83%	144	80	89%	5,750004758	36,68%	100,00%
SR44	88%	180	72	94%	5,325004932	40,56%	100,47%
SR45	91%	216	126	77%	5,133504799	34,45%	104,13%
SR46	86%	260	100	92%	6,944006306	43,46%	95,12%
SR47	88%	216	72	57%	5,499754979	36,17%	107,71%
SR48	62%	228	95	62%	6,680005439	38,94%	101,67%
SR49	85%	228	95	70%	5,41750512	31,75%	96,23%
SR50	94%	240	120	59%	8,907007977	29,20%	90,07%
SR51	84%	190	95	80%	3,795503353	20,47%	71,88%
SR52	88%	247	125	68%	5,968005229	33,80%	93,25%
SR53	93%	378	147	86%	6,229505745	35,74%	96,01%
SR54	48%	190	76	94%	7,145506461	31,64%	110,27%
SR55	90%	228	152	96%	5,234503785	36,79%	102,64%
SR56	82%	220	80	100%	5,368504502	34,58%	101,29%
SR57	86%	171	76	68%	5,198504979	27,11%	78,06%
SR58	94%	228	133	70%	6,577506284	35,23%	97,88%
SR59	88%	240	80	44%	5,724755042	32,32%	118,82%
SR60	63%	180	108	92%	6,352005829	28,73%	85,84%
SR61	83%	260	80	98%	8,105507766	35,49%	100,90%
SR62	90%	220	120	54%	5,95300558	39,27%	118,68%
SR63	90%	260	120	67%	5,46600525	29,46%	90,80%

Table 7.3-1: On the left hand side the data sheet for the fourth quarter 2006 is presented. The columns are headed with an (I) indicating an input dimension and with an (O) for an output dimension.

Quarters	(I)ØF	(I)ØCCD	(I)ØCCP	(I)ØF/T	(O)ØQ	(O)ØSOM/CI	(O)ØTR
Q1 2004	0,79	219	70	0,57	2,59	0,46	0,99
Q2 2004	0,79	209	69	0,63	2,66	0,44	1,40
Q3 2004	0,73	263	95	0,66	2,95	0,45	1,12
Q4 2004	0,88	223	73	0,67	2,83	0,42	0,97
Q1 2005	0,78	209	68	0,43	3,88	0,4	1,27
Q2 2005	0,81	227	84	0,61	4,8	0,38	1,00
Q3 2005	0,79	205	126	0,7	4,58	0,36	1,01
Q4 2005	0,84	214	117	0,76	5,12	0,35	1,10
Q1 2006	0,76	204	105	0,77	5,58	0,33	0,95
Q2 2006	0,82	209	107	0,82	5,84	0,33	1,07
Q3 2006	0,79	267	141	0,8	5,54	0,32	0,91
Q4 2006	0,81	222	102	0,8	6,11	0,32	0,96

Table 7.3-2: The table above depicts the average values of the dimensions over the relevant time interval

7.2.1 Appendix B1 (NO-SBM-V model, Version: F, CCD, CCP, F/T – Q, CI)

DMU	Score	F Inefficiency	CCD Inefficiency	CCP Inefficiency	F/T Inefficiency	Q Inefficiency	CI Inefficiency
SR1	85%	0,0000	0,0000	0,0891	0,0112	0,0526	0,0000
SR2	53%	0,0268	0,0302	0,1310	0,0700	0,2651	0,1438
SR3	58%	0,0000	0,0000	0,1071	0,0184	0,3719	0,1354
SR4	100%	0,0000	0,0000	0,0000	0,0000	0,0000	0,0000
SR5	52%	0,0000	0,0000	0,0141	0,0331	0,5684	0,2601
SR6	100%	0,0000	0,0000	0,0000	0,0000	0,0000	0,0000
SR7	100%	0,0000	0,0000	0,0000	0,0000	0,0000	0,0000
SR8	48%	0,0417	0,0000	0,1875	0,0331	0,4261	0,1266
SR9	83%	0,0060	0,0047	0,1535	0,0000	0,0065	0,0000
SR10	65%	0,0462	0,0278	0,1389	0,0543	0,0861	0,0495
SR11	69%	0,0043	0,0000	0,0500	0,0693	0,0572	0,2110
SR12	92%	0,0000	0,0000	0,0246	0,0278	0,0292	0,0063
SR13	46%	0,0190	0,0000	0,1523	0,0159	0,5593	0,2026
SR14	66%	0,0000	0,0000	0,0775	0,0151	0,3306	0,0451
SR15	100%	0,0000	0,0000	0,0000	0,0000	0,0000	0,0000
SR16	100%	0,0000	0,0000	0,0000	0,0000	0,0000	0,0000
SR17	61%	0,0000	0,0000	0,1023	0,0225	0,3254	0,1113
SR18	64%	0,0000	0,0000	0,0919	0,0394	0,2032	0,1509
SR19	69%	0,0000	0,0000	0,0459	0,0409	0,2036	0,1133
SR20	63%	0,0085	0,0068	0,1270	0,0242	0,3143	0,0000
SR21	61%	0,0121	0,0000	0,0556	0,0511	0,3336	0,1111
SR22	72%	0,0384	0,0000	0,0790	0,0485	0,1361	0,0291
SR23	100%	0,0000	0,0000	0,0000	0,0000	0,0000	0,0000
SR24	65%	0,0000	0,0000	0,1500	0,0522	0,1535	0,0707
SR26	57%	0,0484	0,0244	0,1842	0,0382	0,1630	0,0720
SR27	88%	0,0000	0,0000	0,0259	0,0000	0,0294	0,0800
SR28	67%	0,0163	0,0000	0,1132	0,0220	0,2073	0,0559
SR29	100%	0,0000	0,0000	0,0000	0,0000	0,0000	0,0000
SR30	86%	0,0617	0,0000	0,0762	0,0000	0,0000	0,0000
SR32	100%	0,0000	0,0000	0,0000	0,0000	0,0000	0,0000
SR33	62%	0,0000	0,0000	0,0719	0,0222	0,3415	0,1223
SR34	48%	0,0513	0,0000	0,0984	0,0593	0,6354	0,0000
SR35	56%	0,0000	0,0000	0,0649	0,0090	0,5880	0,0682
SR36	74%	0,0053	0,0000	0,0833	0,0372	0,1779	0,0050
SR37	43%	0,0141	0,0000	0,0625	0,0442	0,7039	0,3309
SR38	75%	0,0000	0,0000	0,0095	0,0371	0,1952	0,0742
SR39	60%	0,0320	0,0357	0,1875	0,0357	0,1758	0,0085
SR40	68%	0,0389	0,0000	0,0903	0,0470	0,1842	0,0212
SR41	59%	0,0320	0,0357	0,1250	0,0278	0,2747	0,0538
SR42	28%	0,0000	0,0000	0,0000	0,0396	2,1755	0,2357
SR43	100%	0,0000	0,0000	0,0000	0,0000	0,0000	0,0000
SR44	100%	0,0000	0,0000	0,0000	0,0000	0,0000	0,0000
SR45	56%	0,0143	0,0000	0,1230	0,0338	0,4585	0,0127
SR46	100%	0,0000	0,0000	0,0000	0,0000	0,0000	0,0000
SR47	100%	0,0000	0,0000	0,0000	0,0000	0,0000	0,0000
SR48	100%	0,0000	0,0000	0,0000	0,0000	0,0000	0,0000
SR49	60%	0,0135	0,0000	0,1132	0,0025	0,3919	0,0612
SR50	80%	0,0055	0,0329	0,0833	0,0000	0,0142	0,0884
SR51	46%	0,0000	0,0000	0,0412	0,0249	0,6782	0,3458
SR52	61%	0,0142	0,0251	0,1414	0,0000	0,3168	0,0249
SR53	50%	0,0484	0,0913	0,1820	0,0407	0,2615	0,0028
SR54	100%	0,0000	0,0000	0,0000	0,0000	0,0000	0,0000
SR55	55%	0,0553	0,0000	0,1506	0,0689	0,3165	0,0000
SR56	61%	0,0000	0,0000	0,0643	0,0779	0,3994	0,0105
SR57	100%	0,0000	0,0000	0,0000	0,0000	0,0000	0,0000
SR58	65%	0,0362	0,0000	0,1523	0,0025	0,2346	0,0056
SR59	100%	0,0000	0,0000	0,0000	0,0000	0,0000	0,0000
SR60	80%	0,0000	0,0000	0,0705	0,0098	0,0676	0,0803
SR61	70%	0,0241	0,0192	0,1250	0,0663	0,0852	0,0064
SR62	100%	0,0000	0,0000	0,0000	0,0000	0,0000	0,0000
SR63	55%	0,0139	0,0406	0,1204	0,0000	0,3978	0,1002

Table 7.2.1-1: The table on the left displays the decomposition of inefficiency for the different sales reps. Each cell depict the contribution to inefficiency for all sales reps who failed to reach the efficiency frontier.

Table 7.2.1-2: The table on the left displays the slacks for the sample

DMU	Excess F S-(1)	Excess CCD S-(2)	Excess CCP S-(3)	Excess F/T S-(4)	Shortage Q S+(1)	Shortage CI S+(2)
SR1	0,00	0,00	42,76	0,04	0,71	0,00
SR2	0,09	33,00	44,00	0,28	3,29	0,08
SR3	0,00	0,00	60,00	0,05	4,30	0,07
SR4	0,00	0,00	0,00	0,00	0,00	0,00
SR5	0,00	0,00	4,53	0,11	4,83	0,12
SR6	0,00	0,00	0,00	0,00	0,00	0,00
SR7	0,00	0,01	0,01	0,00	0,00	0,00
SR8	0,15	0,00	120,00	0,11	4,37	0,07
SR9	0,02	4,49	85,94	0,00	0,11	0,00
SR10	0,17	30,00	50,00	0,20	1,39	0,03
SR11	0,02	0,00	20,00	0,28	0,88	0,11
SR12	0,00	0,00	7,48	0,09	0,46	0,00
SR13	0,07	0,00	81,00	0,05	5,10	0,10
SR14	0,00	0,00	24,81	0,05	3,47	0,03
SR15	0,00	0,00	0,00	0,00	0,00	0,00
SR16	0,00	0,00	0,00	0,00	0,00	0,00
SR17	0,00	0,00	46,66	0,07	3,60	0,06
SR18	0,00	0,00	29,40	0,14	2,50	0,08
SR19	0,00	0,00	17,43	0,16	2,31	0,06
SR20	0,03	7,09	81,26	0,09	3,03	0,00
SR21	0,05	0,00	20,00	0,17	3,97	0,06
SR22	0,15	0,00	24,00	0,17	2,07	0,02
SR23	0,00	0,00	0,00	0,00	0,00	0,00
SR24	0,00	0,00	60,00	0,19	2,23	0,04
SR26	0,18	26,00	112,00	0,13	2,33	0,05
SR27	0,00	0,00	11,17	0,00	0,30	0,04
SR28	0,06	0,00	43,00	0,07	2,83	0,04
SR29	0,00	0,00	0,00	0,00	0,00	0,00
SR30	0,24	0,00	44,82	0,00	0,00	0,00
SR32	0,00	0,00	0,00	0,00	0,00	0,00
SR33	0,00	0,00	28,77	0,08	3,31	0,06
SR34	0,18	0,00	47,22	0,21	4,53	0,00
SR35	0,00	0,00	25,94	0,03	4,74	0,04
SR36	0,02	0,00	40,00	0,11	2,64	0,00
SR37	0,05	0,00	20,00	0,15	5,72	0,14
SR38	0,00	0,00	2,27	0,14	2,25	0,05
SR39	0,11	40,00	120,00	0,12	2,47	0,01
SR40	0,14	0,00	26,00	0,16	2,58	0,01
SR41	0,11	40,00	40,00	0,09	3,36	0,03
SR42	0,00	0,00	0,00	0,13	7,34	0,11
SR43	0,00	0,00	0,00	0,00	0,00	0,00
SR44	0,00	0,00	0,00	0,00	0,00	0,00
SR45	0,05	0,00	62,00	0,10	4,71	0,01
SR46	0,00	0,00	0,00	0,00	0,00	0,00
SR47	0,00	0,00	0,00	0,00	0,00	0,00
SR48	0,00	0,00	0,00	0,00	0,00	0,00
SR49	0,05	0,00	43,00	0,01	4,25	0,04
SR50	0,02	31,58	40,00	0,00	0,25	0,05
SR51	0,00	0,00	15,67	0,08	5,15	0,14
SR52	0,05	24,78	75,23	0,00	3,78	0,02
SR53	0,18	138,00	107,00	0,14	3,26	0,00
SR54	0,00	0,00	0,00	0,00	0,00	0,00
SR55	0,20	0,00	91,59	0,26	3,31	0,00
SR56	0,00	0,00	20,57	0,31	4,29	0,01
SR57	0,00	0,00	0,00	0,00	0,00	0,00
SR58	0,14	0,00	81,00	0,01	3,09	0,00
SR59	0,00	0,00	0,00	0,00	0,00	0,00
SR60	0,00	0,00	30,45	0,04	0,86	0,05
SR61	0,08	20,00	40,00	0,26	1,38	0,00
SR62	0,00	0,00	0,00	0,00	0,00	0,00
SR63	0,05	42,22	57,78	0,00	4,35	0,06

DMU	V(1) F	V(2) CCD	V(3) CCP	V(4) F/T	U(1) Q	U(2) CI
SR1	0,6575	0,0044	0,0021	0,3012	0,0630	2,1515
SR2	0,2976	0,0009	0,0030	0,2500	0,0425	0,9434
SR3	0,2688	0,0017	0,0018	0,3676	0,0502	1,0561
SR4	0,3333	0,0010	0,0063	0,3472	0,0527	1,3911
SR5	0,5614	0,0044	0,0031	0,2941	0,0613	1,1671
SR6	1,1135	0,0011	0,0033	0,3571	0,0771	2,1011
SR7	7,2988	0,0010	0,0025	14,6996	0,7073	1,4752
SR8	0,2778	0,0010	0,0016	0,3012	0,0464	0,8283
SR9	0,3676	0,0010	0,0018	0,8009	0,0503	3,3037
SR10	0,2717	0,0009	0,0028	0,2717	0,0399	0,9865
SR11	0,2747	0,0037	0,0025	0,2500	0,0451	1,3824
SR12	0,5404	0,0045	0,0033	0,2941	0,0587	1,2912
SR13	0,2874	0,0019	0,0019	0,3378	0,0506	0,9098
SR14	0,5656	0,0043	0,0031	0,2976	0,0628	1,0454
SR15	0,2778	0,0852	0,2135	46,8843	0,1177	401,2332
SR16	1,8641	0,0119	0,0025	0,4428	0,2013	7,3720
SR17	0,5534	0,0035	0,0022	0,3086	0,0550	1,0841
SR18	0,5103	0,0041	0,0031	0,2717	0,0522	1,1799
SR19	0,5397	0,0045	0,0026	0,2500	0,0610	1,2868
SR20	0,2941	0,0010	0,0016	0,2660	0,0658	4,8656
SR21	0,2688	0,0028	0,0028	0,3049	0,0512	1,0600
SR22	0,2632	0,0034	0,0033	0,2907	0,0471	1,0630
SR23	0,2841	0,0143	0,0021	0,3425	0,1772	1,6030
SR24	0,3333	0,0010	0,0025	0,2747	0,0449	1,0348
SR26	0,2688	0,0009	0,0016	0,2941	0,0399	0,9082
SR27	1,1297	0,0089	0,0023	1,0543	0,0850	1,6513
SR28	0,2907	0,0027	0,0026	0,3289	0,0492	1,0479
SR29	1,4017	0,0080	0,0028	1,1881	0,1011	1,7477
SR30	0,2577	0,0061	0,0017	1,0989	0,0888	12,6571
SR32	0,2688	0,0027	0,0031	0,3968	0,0777	1,4323
SR33	0,5802	0,0039	0,0025	0,2717	0,0639	1,1662
SR34	0,2907	0,0032	0,0021	0,2809	0,0679	5,5425
SR35	0,6281	0,0038	0,0025	0,3125	0,0694	0,9448
SR36	0,2632	0,0021	0,0021	0,3378	0,0497	1,0692
SR37	0,2809	0,0032	0,0031	0,3049	0,0532	1,0135
SR38	0,4780	0,0051	0,0042	0,2717	0,0650	1,1918
SR39	0,2907	0,0009	0,0016	0,2976	0,0426	0,8472
SR40	0,2717	0,0036	0,0035	0,2874	0,0488	0,9954
SR41	0,2907	0,0009	0,0031	0,3086	0,0479	0,9041
SR42	0,5930	0,0066	0,0056	0,2941	0,0834	0,5902
SR43	0,7340	0,0055	0,0031	0,2809	0,0870	3,8210
SR44	0,2841	0,0048	0,0035	0,2660	0,1218	9,2752
SR45	0,2747	0,0019	0,0020	0,3247	0,0549	0,8179
SR46	0,2907	0,0034	0,0025	0,3738	0,0788	6,9896
SR47	2,6409	0,0012	0,0513	14,8686	0,0909	39,3781
SR48	0,4032	0,0011	0,0026	1,5782	0,1636	12,7085
SR49	0,2941	0,0026	0,0026	0,3571	0,0553	0,9438
SR50	0,2660	0,0010	0,0021	1,3592	0,0447	1,3639
SR51	0,5634	0,0048	0,0026	0,3125	0,0608	1,1271
SR52	0,2841	0,0010	0,0019	0,7224	0,0512	0,9034
SR53	0,2688	0,0007	0,0017	0,2907	0,0405	0,7056
SR54	2,0633	0,0013	0,0033	0,2660	0,1528	2,0507
SR55	0,2778	0,0025	0,0016	0,2604	0,0526	3,8573
SR56	0,4855	0,0041	0,0031	0,2500	0,0567	0,8798
SR57	0,2907	0,0251	0,0168	4,0403	0,0962	1,8441
SR58	0,2660	0,0018	0,0019	0,3571	0,0496	0,9257
SR59	0,2841	0,0010	0,0031	2,7624	0,0873	4,5342
SR60	0,5750	0,0047	0,0023	0,2717	0,0631	1,3942
SR61	0,3012	0,0010	0,0031	0,2551	0,0433	0,9878
SR62	0,2778	0,0063	0,0021	1,1951	0,0840	13,5602
SR63	0,2778	0,0010	0,0021	0,8315	0,0504	0,9348

Table 7.2.1-3: The table on the left displays the individual input and output virtual weights for the sample

DMU	VX(1) F	VX(2) CCD	VX(3) CCP	VX(4) F/T	UY(1) Q	UY(2) CI
SR1	0,41	0,88	0,25	0,25	0,43	0,75
SR2	0,25	0,25	0,25	0,25	0,26	0,26
SR3	0,25	0,34	0,25	0,25	0,29	0,29
SR4	0,25	0,25	0,25	0,25	0,50	0,50
SR5	0,43	0,88	0,25	0,25	0,26	0,26
SR6	0,57	0,25	0,25	0,25	0,50	0,82
SR7	4,74	0,25	0,25	8,82	4,75	0,50
SR8	0,25	0,25	0,25	0,25	0,24	0,24
SR9	0,25	0,25	0,25	0,57	0,42	1,22
SR10	0,25	0,25	0,25	0,25	0,32	0,32
SR11	0,25	0,67	0,25	0,25	0,35	0,35
SR12	0,45	0,86	0,25	0,25	0,46	0,46
SR13	0,25	0,43	0,25	0,25	0,23	0,23
SR14	0,38	0,96	0,25	0,25	0,33	0,33
SR15	0,25	19,42	20,28	37,51	0,50	165,30
SR16	1,21	2,63	0,25	0,30	1,56	2,84
SR17	0,42	0,72	0,25	0,25	0,30	0,30
SR18	0,37	0,91	0,25	0,25	0,32	0,32
SR19	0,35	0,86	0,25	0,25	0,35	0,35
SR20	0,25	0,25	0,25	0,25	0,32	1,99
SR21	0,25	0,59	0,25	0,25	0,31	0,31
SR22	0,25	0,78	0,25	0,25	0,36	0,36
SR23	0,25	2,00	0,25	0,25	1,09	0,50
SR24	0,25	0,25	0,25	0,25	0,33	0,33
SR26	0,25	0,25	0,25	0,25	0,29	0,29
SR27	0,72	1,45	0,25	0,83	0,44	0,44
SR28	0,25	0,63	0,25	0,25	0,34	0,34
SR29	0,62	1,44	0,25	0,94	0,50	0,50
SR30	0,25	1,42	0,25	0,73	0,59	5,03
SR32	0,25	0,53	0,25	0,25	0,78	0,50
SR33	0,36	0,77	0,25	0,25	0,31	0,31
SR34	0,25	0,70	0,25	0,25	0,24	2,06
SR35	0,45	0,77	0,25	0,25	0,28	0,28
SR36	0,25	0,41	0,25	0,25	0,37	0,37
SR37	0,25	0,70	0,25	0,25	0,22	0,22
SR38	0,38	1,01	0,25	0,25	0,38	0,38
SR39	0,25	0,25	0,25	0,25	0,30	0,30
SR40	0,25	0,84	0,25	0,25	0,34	0,34
SR41	0,25	0,25	0,25	0,25	0,29	0,29
SR42	0,50	1,30	0,41	0,25	0,14	0,14
SR43	0,61	0,79	0,25	0,25	0,50	1,40
SR44	0,25	0,86	0,25	0,25	0,65	3,76
SR45	0,25	0,41	0,25	0,25	0,28	0,28
SR46	0,25	0,89	0,25	0,34	0,55	3,04
SR47	2,32	0,25	3,69	8,48	0,50	14,24
SR48	0,25	0,25	0,25	0,98	1,09	4,95
SR49	0,25	0,59	0,25	0,25	0,30	0,30
SR50	0,25	0,25	0,25	0,80	0,40	0,40
SR51	0,47	0,91	0,25	0,25	0,23	0,23
SR52	0,25	0,25	0,25	0,49	0,31	0,31
SR53	0,25	0,25	0,25	0,25	0,25	0,25
SR54	0,99	0,25	0,25	0,25	1,09	0,65
SR55	0,25	0,58	0,25	0,25	0,28	1,42
SR56	0,40	0,91	0,25	0,25	0,30	0,30
SR57	0,25	4,29	1,27	2,75	0,50	0,50
SR58	0,25	0,41	0,25	0,25	0,33	0,33
SR59	0,25	0,25	0,25	1,22	0,50	1,47
SR60	0,36	0,84	0,25	0,25	0,40	0,40
SR61	0,25	0,25	0,25	0,25	0,35	0,35
SR62	0,25	1,38	0,25	0,65	0,50	5,32
SR63	0,25	0,25	0,25	0,56	0,28	0,28

Table 7.2.1-4: The table on the left displays the weighted data set, i.e. the virtual weights times the data of each of the sales rep

Sales Rep	Score	Benchmark	Impact	Benchmark	Impact	Benchmark	Impact	Benchmark	Impact	Benchmark	Impact
SR1	0,85	SR6	0,30	SR32	0,23	SR43	0,08	SR54	0,39		
SR2	0,53	SR4	1,00								
SR3	0,58	SR32	1,00								
SR4	1,00	SR4	1,00								
SR5	0,52	SR4	0,08	SR32	0,60	SR54	0,32				
SR6	1,00	SR6	1,00								
SR7	1,00	SR7	1,00	SR48	0,00						
SR8	0,48	SR4	1,00								
SR9	0,83	SR4	0,63	SR6	0,34	SR48	0,03				
SR10	0,65	SR4	1,00								
SR11	0,69	SR32	0,64	SR43	0,36						
SR12	0,92	SR4	0,29	SR32	0,33	SR43	0,38				
SR13	0,46	SR4	0,70	SR32	0,30						
SR14	0,66	SR4	0,59	SR32	0,07	SR54	0,34				
SR15	1,00	SR15	1,00								
SR16	1,00	SR16	1,00								
SR17	0,61	SR4	0,29	SR32	0,45	SR54	0,26				
SR18	0,64	SR4	0,72	SR43	0,13	SR54	0,15				
SR19	0,69	SR32	0,32	SR43	0,07	SR54	0,61				
SR20	0,63	SR4	0,35	SR46	0,65						
SR21	0,61	SR4	0,25	SR32	0,75						
SR22	0,72	SR4	0,70	SR32	0,30						
SR23	1,00	SR23	1,00								
SR24	0,65	SR4	1,00								
SR26	0,57	SR4	1,00								
SR27	0,88	SR23	0,29	SR29	0,53	SR32	0,00	SR43	0,18		
SR28	0,67	SR4	0,70	SR32	0,30						
SR29	1,00	SR29	1,00								
SR30	0,86	SR16	0,09	SR44	0,00	SR46	0,18	SR48	0,50	SR62	0,23
SR32	1,00	SR32	1,00								
SR33	0,62	SR4	0,16	SR32	0,22	SR54	0,63				
SR34	0,48	SR4	0,13	SR6	0,53	SR32	0,34				
SR35	0,56	SR4	0,11	SR32	0,47	SR54	0,42				
SR36	0,74	SR32	1,00								
SR37	0,43	SR4	0,50	SR32	0,50						
SR38	0,75	SR4	0,56	SR32	0,05	SR43	0,40				
SR39	0,60	SR4	1,00								
SR40	0,68	SR4	0,85	SR32	0,15						
SR41	0,59	SR4	1,00								
SR42	0,28	SR4	0,19	SR32	0,56	SR43	0,16	SR54	0,09		
SR43	1,00	SR43	1,00								
SR44	1,00	SR44	1,00								
SR45	0,56	SR4	0,40	SR32	0,60						
SR46	1,00	SR46	1,00								
SR47	1,00	SR47	1,00								
SR48	1,00	SR48	1,00								
SR49	0,60	SR4	0,70	SR32	0,30						
SR50	0,80	SR32	0,79	SR59	0,21						
SR51	0,46	SR32	0,68	SR43	0,15	SR54	0,17				
SR52	0,61	SR4	0,56	SR32	0,44						
SR53	0,50	SR4	1,00								
SR54	1,00	SR54	1,00								
SR55	0,55	SR4	0,45	SR6	0,35	SR32	0,19				
SR56	0,61	SR4	0,51	SR32	0,45	SR54	0,04				
SR57	1,00	SR32	0,00	SR57	1,00						
SR58	0,65	SR4	0,70	SR32	0,30						
SR59	1,00	SR59	1,00								
SR60	0,80	SR32	0,14	SR43	0,25	SR54	0,61				
SR61	0,70	SR4	1,00								
SR62	1,00	SR62	1,00								
SR63	0,55	SR4	0,44	SR32	0,56						

Table 7.2.1-5: The table on the left displays the individual benchmark partners for inefficient sales reps for the SBM model version 1 (remember: Returns to Scale = Variable (Sum of Lambda = 1))

Sales Rep	Score	Benchmark	Impact	Benchmark	Impact	Benchmark	Impact	Benchmark	Impact	Benchmark	Impact
SR1	0,85	SR6	0,30	SR32	0,23	SR43	0,08	SR54	0,39		
SR2	0,53	SR4	1,00								
SR3	0,58	SR32	1,00								
SR4	1,00	SR4	1,00								
SR5	0,52	SR4	0,08	SR32	0,60	SR54	0,32				
SR6	1,00	SR6	1,00								
SR7	1,00	SR7	1,00	SR48	0,00						
SR8	0,48	SR4	1,00								
SR9	0,83	SR4	0,63	SR6	0,34	SR48	0,03				
SR10	0,65	SR4	1,00								
SR11	0,69	SR32	0,64	SR43	0,36						
SR12	0,92	SR4	0,29	SR32	0,33	SR43	0,38				
SR13	0,46	SR4	0,70	SR32	0,30						
SR14	0,66	SR4	0,59	SR32	0,07	SR54	0,34				
SR15	1,00	SR15	1,00								
SR16	1,00	SR16	1,00								
SR17	0,61	SR4	0,29	SR32	0,45	SR54	0,26				
SR18	0,64	SR4	0,72	SR43	0,13	SR54	0,15				
SR19	0,69	SR32	0,32	SR43	0,07	SR54	0,61				
SR20	0,63	SR4	0,35	SR46	0,65						
SR21	0,61	SR4	0,25	SR32	0,75						
SR22	0,72	SR4	0,70	SR32	0,30						
SR23	1,00	SR23	1,00								
SR24	0,65	SR4	1,00								
SR26	0,57	SR4	1,00								
SR27	0,88	SR23	0,29	SR29	0,53	SR32	0,00	SR43	0,18		
SR28	0,67	SR4	0,70	SR32	0,30						
SR29	1,00	SR29	1,00								
SR30	0,86	SR16	0,09	SR44	0,00	SR46	0,18	SR48	0,50	SR62	0,23
SR32	1,00	SR32	1,00								
SR33	0,62	SR4	0,16	SR32	0,22	SR54	0,63				
SR34	0,48	SR4	0,13	SR6	0,53	SR32	0,34				
SR35	0,56	SR4	0,11	SR32	0,47	SR54	0,42				
SR36	0,74	SR32	1,00								
SR37	0,43	SR4	0,50	SR32	0,50						
SR38	0,75	SR4	0,56	SR32	0,05	SR43	0,40				
SR39	0,60	SR4	1,00								
SR40	0,68	SR4	0,85	SR32	0,15						
SR41	0,59	SR4	1,00								
SR42	0,28	SR4	0,19	SR32	0,56	SR43	0,16	SR54	0,09		
SR43	1,00	SR43	1,00								
SR44	1,00	SR44	1,00								
SR45	0,56	SR4	0,40	SR32	0,60						
SR46	1,00	SR46	1,00								
SR47	1,00	SR47	1,00								
SR48	1,00	SR48	1,00								
SR49	0,60	SR4	0,70	SR32	0,30						
SR50	0,80	SR32	0,79	SR59	0,21						
SR51	0,46	SR32	0,68	SR43	0,15	SR54	0,17				
SR52	0,61	SR4	0,56	SR32	0,44						
SR53	0,50	SR4	1,00								
SR54	1,00	SR54	1,00								
SR55	0,55	SR4	0,45	SR6	0,35	SR32	0,19				
SR56	0,61	SR4	0,51	SR32	0,45	SR54	0,04				
SR57	1,00	SR32	0,00	SR57	1,00						
SR58	0,65	SR4	0,70	SR32	0,30						
SR59	1,00	SR59	1,00								
SR60	0,80	SR32	0,14	SR43	0,25	SR54	0,61				
SR61	0,70	SR4	1,00								
SR62	1,00	SR62	1,00								
SR63	0,55	SR4	0,44	SR32	0,56						

Table 7.2.1-6: The table on the left displays the status quo value for q4 2006 and the optimized target values for the SBM model version 1

Sales Rep	q1 2004	q2 2004	q3 2004	q4 2004	q1 2005	q2 2005	q3 2005	q4 2005	q1 2006	q2 2006	q3 2006	q4 2006
SR1	0,60	0,53	0,55	5,64	0,60	0,62	0,69	0,67	0,64	0,60	0,77	0,85
SR2	0,62	0,79	0,67	1,12	0,66	0,51	0,58	0,56	0,67	0,66	0,59	0,53
SR3	0,40	0,41	0,56	1,12	0,77	0,60	1,07	1,03	1,02	0,70	0,65	0,58
SR4	0,52	0,53	0,84	1,10	0,79	0,65	0,73	0,86	1,04	1,05	1,03	1,29
SR5	1,00	1,02	1,17	1,08	0,45	0,44	0,51	0,38	0,61	0,48	0,57	0,52
SR6	1,06	1,11	1,08	1,05	1,02	1,24	0,87	1,02	0,76	0,72	1,03	1,09
SR7	0,41	0,60	0,64	1,05	0,61	1,00	1,02	0,45	1,05	1,05	1,07	1,00
SR8	1,00	0,56	0,61	1,04	0,63	1,15	0,64	0,57	0,54	0,47	0,56	0,48
SR9	1,00	1,00	1,00	1,03	1,01	1,01	1,01	0,92	0,90	0,84	1,00	0,83
SR10	0,68	0,72	0,87	1,03	0,78	0,58	0,60	0,62	0,76	0,52	0,60	0,65
SR11	1,17	1,00	0,77	1,02	1,09	0,61	1,03	1,07	0,64	0,63	0,69	0,69
SR12	0,43	0,66	1,27	1,01	1,45	1,38	1,04	1,02	1,05	0,68	0,89	0,92
SR13	0,48	0,52	0,73	1,00	0,65	0,58	0,84	0,69	0,50	0,42	0,65	0,46
SR14	0,42	0,62	0,78	1,00	0,61	0,41	0,48	0,46	0,73	0,59	0,82	0,66
SR15	0,60	0,65	1,06	0,92	0,62	1,02	0,51	1,00	0,62	0,63	0,65	1,00
SR16	1,02	0,70	0,75	0,78	0,80	0,66	1,03	0,93	0,96	0,93	1,01	1,01
SR17	0,50	0,60	0,62	0,78	1,06	0,47	0,51	11,47	0,66	0,57	0,56	0,61
SR18	0,61	0,60	1,04	0,77	0,77	0,61	1,23	1,00	1,03	0,51	0,67	0,64
SR19	1,02	0,57	1,11	0,76	1,02	0,51	1,00	0,49	0,51	0,44	0,50	0,69
SR20	0,44	0,50	0,61	0,75	0,56	0,35	0,42	0,53	0,66	0,49	0,40	0,63
SR21	0,58	0,46	0,58	0,75	0,74	0,58	0,51	0,59	0,53	0,52	0,62	0,61
SR22	0,87	1,00	1,08	0,74	1,10	0,56	0,67	0,80	1,05	0,83	0,71	0,72
SR23	0,42	0,44	0,77	0,71	1,02	0,61	0,79	0,62	1,04	0,74	0,72	1,05
SR24	0,48	0,55	0,55	0,71	0,77	1,01	0,80	0,73	0,93	0,75	0,68	0,65
SR26	0,37	0,56	1,00	0,66	0,70	0,64	0,63	1,01	0,54	0,42	0,53	0,57
SR27	0,30	0,44	0,53	0,65	0,55	0,36	0,50	0,58	0,61	0,55	0,58	0,88
SR28	0,70	0,51	0,70	0,64	1,01	0,54	0,70	0,76	0,83	0,67	0,75	0,67
SR29	0,49	1,06	0,65	0,64	0,62	0,52	0,77	1,01	0,65	0,57	0,73	1,08
SR30	0,75	0,55	0,68	0,63	0,70	0,53	0,64	0,75	0,88	0,70	0,66	0,86
SR32	1,12	1,20	1,05	0,63	0,58	0,64	0,63	0,60	1,11	1,06	1,12	1,12
SR33	1,05	0,62	1,00	0,63	0,74	0,35	0,50	0,41	0,54	0,53	0,49	0,62
SR34	0,47	0,51	0,54	0,63	0,56	0,43	0,56	0,61	0,60	0,46	0,47	0,48
SR35	0,60	0,63	0,82	0,62	0,67	0,65	1,14	1,09	1,56	0,56	2,10	0,56
SR36	1,03	1,04	1,05	0,61	1,08	1,03	1,11	1,14	1,01	0,80	0,75	0,74
SR37	1,00	0,55	0,59	0,61	0,78	0,50	1,02	1,00	0,53	1,00	0,51	0,43
SR38	0,36	0,46	0,46	0,61	0,59	0,40	0,50	0,37	0,61	0,49	0,54	0,75
SR39	0,79	0,64	1,07	0,60	0,72	0,64	0,82	0,77	1,01	0,76	0,77	0,60
SR40	1,01	1,51	1,06	0,58	0,62	1,01	1,02	0,55	0,80	0,63	0,76	0,68
SR41	0,68	1,02	1,00	0,58	0,75	0,51	0,70	0,66	1,06	0,65	0,64	0,59
SR42	0,34	0,49	0,67	0,58	0,46	0,38	0,57	0,41	0,27	1,11	0,28	0,28
SR43	1,08	1,06	1,01	0,57	1,08	0,53	1,00	1,01	0,78	0,62	0,72	1,05
SR44	0,47	0,54	1,01	0,57	0,74	0,55	0,74	0,79	0,67	0,67	0,79	1,04
SR45	0,32	0,42	0,42	0,57	0,53	0,43	0,62	0,54	0,66	0,51	0,60	0,56
SR46	0,65	0,58	0,95	0,56	0,80	1,05	1,16	1,09	1,13	1,10	1,09	1,05
SR47	0,50	0,52	0,60	0,56	0,62	0,43	0,53	0,53	0,64	1,01	0,77	1,04
SR48	1,11	1,20	1,21	0,56	1,08	1,00	1,05	1,06	1,05	1,06	1,07	1,02
SR49	1,10	1,10	1,30	0,53	1,00	0,56	0,49	0,67	0,69	0,53	0,68	0,60
SR50	0,57	0,55	0,69	0,51	1,14	1,05	1,02	1,03	1,02	1,02	1,07	0,80
SR51	0,30	0,43	0,55	0,51	0,58	0,48	0,58	0,57	0,49	0,49	0,58	0,46
SR52	0,78	0,59	1,01	0,50	0,78	1,03	1,08	0,78	0,78	0,85	1,00	0,61
SR53	1,02	0,51	0,48	0,49	0,81	0,58	0,72	0,85	1,07	1,41	0,52	0,50
SR54	1,00	0,54	0,39	0,48	0,66	0,55	0,54	0,41	0,79	0,59	1,06	1,08
SR55	0,45	0,52	0,57	0,48	0,65	0,48	0,51	0,49	0,63	0,49	0,44	0,55
SR56	1,05	1,04	1,13	0,48	1,04	0,32	0,42	1,01	0,64	0,60	0,71	0,61
SR57	0,81	0,64	0,66	0,46	1,09	0,46	0,55	0,49	0,79	0,68	0,61	1,03
SR58	0,58	0,62	0,73	0,46	1,05	0,54	0,73	0,63	0,79	0,71	0,81	0,65
SR59	0,52	0,49	0,66	0,45	0,62	0,49	0,50	0,64	1,02	0,81	1,02	1,07
SR60	0,56	0,46	0,59	0,42	0,67	0,51	0,74	0,73	0,73	0,70	0,72	0,80
SR61	0,26	0,33	0,38	0,42	0,45	0,44	0,54	0,53	0,60	0,58	0,60	0,70
SR62	0,71	0,70	0,77	0,40	0,84	0,59	0,69	0,66	0,74	0,72	0,80	1,05
SR63	0,33	0,55	1,40	0,40	0,69	0,57	0,56	0,66	0,72	0,51	0,64	0,55

Table 7.2.1-7: The table on the left displays the efficiency scores over time from q1 2004 to q4 2006 calculated with the NO-*Super*-SBM-V model. If the data is processed with the NO-SBM-V model the only difference is that the efficiency scores exceeding unity are bounded to unity. All the other scores remain unchanged.

Catch up	q12004=> q22004	q22004=> q32004	q32004=> q42004	q42004=> q12005	q12005=> q22005	q22005=> q32005	q32005=> q42005	q42005=> q12006	q12006=> q22006	q22006=> q32006	q32006=> q42006	Ø
SR1	0,8200	1,0421	1,0520	1,0675	1,0302	1,0671	0,9954	0,9005	0,9540	1,2530	1,1859	1,03
SR2	0,8513	1,0460	0,9679	0,9858	0,8148	1,1620	1,0527	1,1401	1,0265	0,8474	0,9688	0,99
SR3	0,9732	1,4731	0,8981	1,5069	0,7557	1,7005	0,9656	0,9662	0,7148	0,9323	0,9650	1,08
SR4	0,9634	1,6542	0,9293	0,9703	0,9168	1,0528	1,2143	1,1802	0,9708	0,9580	1,0652	1,08
SR5	1,0000	1,1137	0,9012	0,4565	1,0701	1,0980	0,9913	1,0391	0,8533	1,1576	0,9484	0,97
SR6	1,0035	0,9417	1,0169	0,9857	1,1432	0,7587	1,0689	0,8311	0,9026	1,1119	1,3637	1,01
SR7	1,2137	1,2196	0,9615	0,8228	1,9087	1,0243	0,5642	1,8108	1,0161	1,0335	0,9132	1,14
SR8	0,5447	1,2262	1,0278	0,9105	1,8177	0,5480	1,0805	0,8456	0,9120	1,1285	0,9429	1,00
SR9	1,0000	0,8258	1,0172	1,2131	0,9892	1,0042	0,9521	0,9644	0,9556	1,1328	0,9585	1,00
SR10	0,8406	1,4179	0,8023	1,1873	0,8279	0,9938	1,2167	0,9678	0,7785	1,0276	1,2451	1,03
SR11	0,6026	1,1581	1,1197	1,2328	0,5612	1,1592	1,7548	0,5021	1,0601	1,0395	1,0478	1,02
SR12	1,6344	1,9335	0,8631	0,9103	1,0291	0,6547	1,3147	1,1615	0,6725	1,2784	0,9839	1,13
SR13	0,9436	1,5000	0,8277	1,0285	0,9354	1,3119	0,9146	0,7158	0,8497	1,6533	0,7043	1,03
SR14	1,1774	1,5308	0,6810	1,1946	0,6996	1,0759	1,0976	1,2997	0,9130	1,3428	0,8248	1,08
SR15	1,0838	1,5459	0,6162	1,1245	1,4768	0,5157	1,9162	0,5939	1,0921	0,9375	1,2709	1,11
SR16	0,7592	1,0303	1,0356	1,0273	0,8525	1,1669	1,1323	0,9467	1,0272	1,0919	0,9973	1,01
SR17	0,9861	1,1890	0,9263	1,8317	0,4493	0,9889	1,3620	0,8583	0,8921	1,0053	1,3156	1,07
SR18	0,9674	1,6053	0,9847	0,7896	0,8545	1,8534	0,7934	0,8153	0,6340	1,3203	0,9503	1,05
SR19	0,6048	1,8404	0,9337	0,9552	0,5926	1,6574	0,6823	0,7686	0,9168	1,1150	1,3336	1,04
SR20	0,9812	1,3446	0,7965	1,1262	0,6579	1,1630	1,2615	1,1614	0,8065	0,8025	1,5875	1,06
SR21	0,7882	1,2931	0,9975	1,3418	0,8575	0,8489	1,1939	0,8247	0,9392	1,2037	0,9920	1,03
SR22	1,1253	1,0977	0,6088	1,6267	0,5322	1,1119	1,3325	1,0429	0,9099	0,8903	1,0059	1,03
SR23	0,9261	1,8590	0,6347	1,6821	0,6927	1,1016	0,9404	1,5798	0,7398	1,0235	1,3391	1,14
SR24	0,9193	1,1288	1,0975	1,1695	1,4007	0,7257	1,0626	1,0410	0,9408	0,8846	1,0929	1,04
SR26	1,2920	1,1577	3,5043	0,3599	0,9387	0,9024	1,6322	0,5403	0,8323	1,1614	1,2411	1,23
SR27	1,2139	1,2562	1,0271	1,1204	0,6537	1,3120	1,2111	1,0048	0,9631	1,0571	1,4262	1,11
SR28	0,6594	1,2923	1,1361	1,3178	0,5918	1,1758	1,1951	0,9549	0,8792	1,0453	0,9940	1,02
SR29	1,9387	0,6295	0,9954	0,9820	0,8834	1,3524	1,3078	0,5974	0,9345	1,3380	1,4333	1,13
SR30	0,6998	1,3317	1,0387	0,9349	0,8095	1,0179	1,3026	1,0579	0,8549	0,9375	1,3511	1,03
SR32	1,0659	0,8558	0,6637	0,8244	1,1040	1,0289	0,9558	1,6966	0,9865	1,0548	1,0234	1,02
SR33	0,6323	1,5132	0,7461	0,8963	0,5741	1,3496	1,0104	0,9528	1,0716	0,9099	1,3451	1,00
SR34	1,0362	1,1051	0,9887	0,8737	0,8129	1,2318	1,1114	0,9686	0,7852	0,9626	1,0618	1,00
SR35	1,0477	1,2673	0,9850	0,8179	1,0489	1,5211	1,0024	1,4685	0,3496	3,5501	0,2915	1,21
SR36	1,0099	1,0092	1,0701	0,9658	0,9493	1,0647	1,0074	0,9164	0,8577	0,9685	0,9486	0,98
SR37	0,5350	1,2010	1,0686	1,0692	0,7484	1,2495	1,0324	0,6234	0,8732	1,2518	0,9179	0,96
SR38	1,0934	1,1483	1,0235	1,0936	0,7803	1,1359	1,0066	1,1344	0,8735	1,0985	1,2802	1,06
SR39	0,8722	1,4998	0,7170	1,0072	0,9127	1,1555	1,0417	1,1894	0,8360	0,9954	0,8390	1,01
SR40	0,8360	1,2084	0,9882	0,5887	1,7186	0,9885	0,6366	1,2839	0,7939	1,0628	1,0186	1,01
SR41	0,9273	1,0511	1,0709	1,0814	0,7650	1,2034	1,0694	0,9706	0,9743	1,0155	0,9524	1,01
SR42	1,2283	1,4068	0,8234	0,8284	0,8269	1,3669	1,0836	0,4554	4,1377	0,2289	1,0411	1,22
SR43	0,9563	0,5335	0,7946	2,4781	0,5081	1,0200	1,2594	1,1520	0,7847	1,1402	1,4869	1,10
SR44	1,0606	1,7522	1,0850	0,6932	0,7772	1,2448	1,4117	0,6820	1,0252	1,1608	1,2079	1,10
SR45	1,0626	1,1473	1,0020	1,1361	0,9069	1,3198	1,0472	1,0676	0,8022	1,0472	1,0811	1,06
SR46	0,8977	1,5870	0,8462	0,9899	1,2874	1,1132	0,9482	0,9999	0,9919	0,9952	0,9566	1,06
SR47	0,9841	1,1100	0,9847	1,0476	0,7762	1,0692	1,1708	1,0885	1,5212	0,7810	1,0422	1,05
SR48	1,0690	1,0167	0,9404	0,9708	0,9461	1,0294	1,0316	1,0048	0,9927	1,0210	0,9455	1,00
SR49	0,9961	1,2355	0,4420	1,6143	0,6671	0,7167	1,3853	1,0023	0,8464	1,2291	0,9501	1,01
SR50	0,8948	1,3272	1,4370	0,9657	1,0335	0,9702	1,0087	0,9984	0,9986	1,0296	0,8158	1,04
SR51	1,2227	1,3892	0,7719	1,3336	0,9098	1,1175	1,0754	0,7426	0,9855	1,2587	0,8043	1,06
SR52	0,7339	1,6539	0,9403	0,8318	1,3103	1,0681	0,6994	0,9939	1,1257	1,1578	0,6890	1,02
SR53	0,4880	1,0205	1,3275	1,1446	0,7957	1,1000	1,2371	1,2952	1,3049	0,3809	1,0817	1,02
SR54	0,4889	0,8391	1,1206	1,3469	0,9549	0,9025	1,0661	1,3232	0,7953	1,8080	1,0255	1,06
SR55	1,0956	1,0776	1,0312	1,0527	0,8467	0,9691	1,2406	1,0516	0,8351	0,8594	1,3512	1,04
SR56	0,9826	1,1331	0,8581	0,1504	0,3131	1,2364	2,4922	0,6239	0,9612	0,9569	1,0711	1,06
SR57	1,3641	0,9774	0,8178	2,0226	0,4355	1,1626	1,1022	1,1842	0,9060	0,9203	1,2271	1,10
SR58	0,9780	1,1905	0,9591	1,5552	0,5569	1,2546	0,9857	1,1315	0,9321	1,1902	0,8726	1,05
SR59	0,8915	1,4227	0,9959	0,9093	0,8694	0,8711	1,2703	1,3775	0,9249	1,3099	1,0534	1,08
SR60	0,8162	1,2273	1,1019	0,9870	0,8414	1,3791	0,9733	1,0039	0,8949	1,1086	1,1205	1,04
SR61	1,0399	1,2185	1,0770	1,1363	1,0462	1,1367	1,1286	1,0417	0,9453	0,9324	1,3620	1,10
SR62	0,8941	1,1237	0,8862	1,1817	0,7816	1,0808	1,0240	1,0384	0,9967	1,0419	1,3003	1,03
SR63	1,3494	2,2311	0,4650	1,2237	1,0319	0,9540	1,1565	1,1345	0,7408	1,1641	0,9470	1,13
Ø	0,9683	1,2650	0,9760	1,1079	0,8948	1,1068	1,1341	1,0116	0,9638	1,1017	1,0747	1,05
Max	1,9387	2,2311	3,5043	2,4781	1,9087	1,8534	2,4922	1,8108	4,1377	3,5501	1,5875	1,23
Min	0,4880	0,5335	0,4420	0,3599	0,3131	0,5157	0,5642	0,4554	0,3496	0,2289	0,2915	0,96
SD	0,2534	0,3058	0,3748	0,3443	0,3084	0,2433	0,2905	0,2679	0,4414	0,3913	0,2232	0,06

Table 7.2.1-8: The catch up process of the individual sales reps

Fronti er	q12004=> q22004	q22004=> q32004	q32004=> q42004	q42004=> q12005	q12005=> q22005	q22005=> q32005	q32005=> q42005	q42005=> q12006	q12006=> q22006	q22006=> q32006	q32006=> q42006	Ø
SR1	1,1159	0,8789	0,8982	1,4382	1,3125	0,8572	0,7962	1,1267	1,0878	0,7876	1,0959	1,04
SR2	1,1889	0,8212	0,7632	1,5169	1,1838	0,8158	0,9018	1,0370	1,0089	0,8492	1,0613	1,01
SR3	0,9507	0,7408	0,9209	1,4665	1,1795	0,5954	0,8740	0,8812	0,9845	0,9142	1,1385	0,97
SR4	1,0336	0,7761	0,8813	1,3950	1,2999	0,9108	0,7817	1,0426	1,0098	1,0026	1,0488	1,02
SR5	1,0957	1,0617	0,7125	1,6483	1,1181	0,8804	0,8612	1,1353	1,0792	0,7974	1,0668	1,04
SR6	1,0329	1,0409	0,8563	1,3094	1,0053	0,9282	0,8500	1,0684	1,0014	0,8361	1,0636	1,00
SR7	0,9152	0,7834	0,7612	1,5204	1,2181	1,0553	0,8537	1,1164	0,9391	1,0013	1,0358	1,02
SR8	1,0254	0,8416	0,9191	1,5031	1,1194	0,2956	0,8729	1,0930	1,0534	0,8423	1,0731	0,97
SR9	1,0000	0,9538	0,8609	1,2408	1,1740	1,1324	0,9411	1,1210	0,9573	0,9514	1,1001	1,04
SR10	1,1233	1,0740	0,8183	1,4314	1,2119	0,8275	0,8803	1,1018	1,0116	0,8706	1,0643	1,04
SR11	1,1078	0,8563	1,0457	1,3362	1,4411	0,8951	0,8707	1,1478	1,0636	0,7316	1,2614	1,07
SR12	1,0832	0,7361	0,9705	1,3865	0,9896	0,9183	0,7775	1,0783	1,0453	0,7887	1,1326	0,99
SR13	0,9657	0,7758	0,8569	1,4434	1,1573	0,8054	0,8438	1,0702	1,0435	1,0372	1,1444	1,01
SR14	0,8980	0,7425	0,8491	1,5168	1,1533	0,8101	0,6538	1,2826	1,0481	0,9959	1,1162	1,01
SR15	1,0092	0,9127	0,9392	1,1829	0,6638	0,9580	0,8698	1,8238	1,0148	0,7528	0,9526	1,01
SR16	1,3616	0,9080	0,9326	1,3012	1,2922	0,9007	0,9631	1,0850	0,9592	0,9558	1,0674	1,07
SR17	0,9729	0,6760	0,9462	1,4984	1,0742	0,8618	0,8738	1,1148	1,0917	0,8050	1,0795	1,00
SR18	1,1838	0,9366	0,9811	1,4900	1,1402	0,8518	0,8396	1,2550	0,9945	0,7823	1,0830	1,05
SR19	1,2961	0,5166	1,0304	1,4750	1,0475	0,9980	0,8876	1,1738	1,0369	0,7825	1,0561	1,03
SR20	1,0163	0,8038	0,7940	1,5160	1,1298	0,8827	0,8833	1,1639	1,0104	0,8626	1,0447	1,01
SR21	0,9697	0,8715	0,9001	1,3517	1,3393	0,8159	0,8801	1,1234	1,0634	0,8892	1,0986	1,03
SR22	1,1176	1,1065	0,9000	1,3755	1,1255	0,8666	0,8633	1,1644	1,0369	0,8386	1,0985	1,04
SR23	0,9399	0,9552	0,8437	1,3854	1,0971	0,8275	0,8851	1,0666	1,0171	0,8384	1,0697	0,99
SR24	1,0092	0,7927	0,9410	1,4586	1,1247	1,1247	0,8143	1,0846	0,9732	0,8805	1,0655	1,02
SR26	0,9974	0,5745	0,7215	1,2452	1,3501	0,9172	0,9320	1,2685	1,0488	0,8825	1,0686	1,00
SR27	0,8970	0,7756	0,9504	1,5626	1,0710	0,8747	0,8653	1,3402	1,0585	0,8278	0,9666	1,02
SR28	1,1107	0,8474	0,9607	1,3983	1,2810	0,8254	0,8674	1,0864	0,9853	0,8998	1,1075	1,03
SR29	1,0359	1,0446	0,7856	1,4821	1,0991	0,7579	0,7574	1,3154	1,0324	1,0821	1,0532	1,04
SR30	1,0760	0,8935	0,8457	1,3432	1,1783	0,8646	0,7298	1,1469	0,9836	0,9578	1,0924	1,01
SR32	0,9771	1,0520	1,0596	0,9483	1,0791	0,8320	0,9417	0,9377	1,0502	0,9553	1,0554	0,99
SR33	1,1904	0,9562	1,1486	1,5050	0,8553	0,8178	0,8823	1,1073	1,0818	0,8189	1,0448	1,04
SR34	1,0233	0,8065	0,9404	1,3086	1,1813	0,8501	0,8758	1,1227	1,0356	0,8647	1,0828	1,01
SR35	1,1906	1,0337	0,8809	1,3681	1,2200	0,8383	0,9098	1,0518	1,1156	0,7547	1,1110	1,04
SR36	1,2515	0,9836	1,0353	1,0993	1,2383	1,0196	1,0237	1,0330	1,2058	0,8649	1,1821	1,09
SR37	1,0282	0,8320	0,8924	1,4064	1,1167	0,9369	0,7501	1,1498	1,0974	0,7882	1,1065	1,01
SR38	0,9194	0,7259	0,9449	1,3948	1,1186	0,8392	0,8853	1,1418	1,0892	0,8461	1,0599	1,00
SR39	1,3751	0,9711	0,9241	1,3578	1,3271	0,8208	0,8627	0,9969	0,9964	0,8674	1,0670	1,05
SR40	0,8477	0,9945	0,8636	1,1568	1,0730	1,0135	0,8574	1,1351	1,0242	0,8621	1,0922	0,99
SR41	1,1343	0,7933	0,9284	1,4288	1,1347	0,8269	0,8675	1,1162	1,0466	0,8408	1,0737	1,02
SR42	0,9151	0,7475	0,8839	1,4425	1,1173	0,8704	0,6853	1,1441	1,0054	1,0042	1,1124	0,99
SR43	1,0210	1,3544	0,7046	1,0830	1,1011	0,8742	0,8180	1,1193	1,0331	0,7965	1,0223	0,99
SR44	1,0162	0,9677	0,9581	1,1720	1,1856	0,8930	0,9158	1,2980	1,0392	0,7464	1,0377	1,02
SR45	0,9063	0,8204	0,9343	1,3444	1,1159	0,8303	0,8944	1,0755	1,0238	0,8846	1,1038	0,99
SR46	1,0791	0,9547	0,9001	1,2951	1,0592	0,9870	0,8917	1,1303	1,0108	0,8632	1,0115	1,02
SR47	1,4006	0,8295	0,9104	1,4862	1,1472	0,8165	0,8883	1,0996	0,9935	0,9405	1,1951	1,06
SR48	1,1481	0,9590	0,9538	1,0728	1,0012	0,8263	0,9619	0,9913	0,9550	0,9740	1,0476	0,99
SR49	0,9992	1,0570	0,9745	0,7728	1,1491	0,7482	0,8739	1,1032	1,0226	0,9141	1,1132	0,98
SR50	1,0887	0,6823	0,8193	1,5080	1,1690	0,9611	1,0681	1,0999	0,9741	0,9851	1,2160	1,05
SR51	0,9144	0,8430	0,9101	1,4284	1,1375	0,8400	0,8695	1,1364	1,1222	0,8426	1,1261	1,02
SR52	1,1638	0,7903	0,9269	1,4040	1,0719	0,7986	0,9051	1,2294	1,0220	0,8280	1,2359	1,03
SR53	1,0337	0,8043	0,9594	1,2745	1,4088	0,8565	0,9205	1,1192	0,9110	0,9940	1,0260	1,03
SR54	1,0418	0,8147	0,9540	1,4902	1,1289	0,8442	0,8650	1,2647	1,0859	0,8763	1,0302	1,04
SR55	0,9679	0,8442	0,9388	1,3154	1,1286	0,8892	0,8681	1,1258	1,0822	0,8734	1,0885	1,01
SR56	0,9935	0,8467	1,0715	0,9808	1,1087	0,9613	0,6345	1,0424	1,0914	0,8244	1,0811	0,97
SR57	0,7225	0,9665	1,1165	0,7662	1,0380	0,8540	0,8729	1,2420	0,8570	0,9167	1,0594	0,95
SR58	1,1412	0,8832	0,9469	1,2804	1,1193	0,8299	0,8737	1,1000	1,0074	0,9048	1,1163	1,02
SR59	1,0452	0,7504	0,7914	1,5571	1,1768	0,8031	0,9311	0,9906	0,9293	0,9481	1,2121	1,01
SR60	1,2384	0,8963	0,8616	1,5321	1,1441	0,8285	0,8210	1,1864	1,2721	0,6998	1,0268	1,05
SR61	0,9242	0,8485	0,9909	1,3506	1,1413	0,8942	0,8686	1,1185	1,0374	0,8836	1,0611	1,01
SR62	1,1665	0,8237	0,8706	1,3974	1,1096	0,9031	0,7815	1,1066	0,9823	0,9192	1,0202	1,01
SR63	1,0029	0,9778	0,8679	1,6096	1,1076	0,8437	0,8867	1,2301	1,0336	0,8352	1,0973	1,04
Ø	1,0557	0,8739	0,9090	1,3567	1,1438	0,8656	0,8627	1,1354	1,0318	0,8748	1,0856	1,02
Max	1,4006	1,3544	1,1486	1,6483	1,4411	1,1324	1,0681	1,8238	1,2721	1,0821	1,2614	1,09
Min	0,7225	0,5166	0,7046	0,7662	0,6638	0,2956	0,6345	0,8812	0,8570	0,6998	0,9526	0,95
SD	0,1288	0,1358	0,0903	0,1818	0,1189	0,1132	0,0741	0,1245	0,0642	0,0805	0,0576	0,03

Table 7.2.1-9: The frontier shift of the individual sales reps

Malm quist	q12004=> q22004	q22004=> q32004	q32004=> q42004	q42004=> q12005	q12005=> q22005	q22005=> q32005	q32005=> q42005	q42005=> q12006	q12006=> q22006	q22006=> q32006	q32006=> q42006	Ø
SR1	0,9150	0,9160	0,9449	1,5353	1,3521	0,9147	0,7925	1,0146	1,0378	0,9869	1,2997	1,06
SR2	1,0121	0,8589	0,7387	1,4954	0,9646	0,9480	0,9493	1,1823	1,0356	0,7196	1,0281	0,99
SR3	0,9252	1,0912	0,8271	2,2098	0,8913	1,0124	0,8439	0,8513	0,7037	0,8522	1,0987	1,03
SR4	0,9958	1,2839	0,8190	1,3536	1,1918	0,9589	0,9493	1,2305	0,9803	0,9605	1,1171	1,08
SR5	1,0957	1,1825	0,6421	0,7525	1,1965	0,9667	0,8538	1,1797	0,9209	0,9231	1,0118	0,98
SR6	1,0366	0,9802	0,8707	1,2907	1,1493	0,7042	0,9086	0,8880	0,9038	0,9296	1,4505	1,01
SR7	1,1107	0,9555	0,7319	1,2510	2,3250	1,0810	0,4817	2,0216	0,9542	1,0348	0,9459	1,17
SR8	0,5586	1,0320	0,9447	1,3686	2,0347	0,1620	0,9432	0,9242	0,9607	0,9505	1,0119	0,99
SR9	1,0000	0,7876	0,8756	1,5053	1,1614	1,1372	0,8960	1,0811	0,9148	1,0777	1,0544	1,04
SR10	0,9443	1,5228	0,6565	1,6995	1,0033	0,8223	1,0710	1,0664	0,7875	0,8946	1,3252	1,07
SR11	0,6675	0,9917	1,1708	1,6474	0,8087	1,0376	1,5279	0,5763	1,1275	0,7606	1,3217	1,06
SR12	1,7704	1,4232	0,8377	1,2621	1,0184	0,6013	1,0222	1,2524	0,7030	1,0083	1,1143	1,09
SR13	0,9112	1,1637	0,7093	1,4846	1,0826	1,0567	0,7717	0,7660	0,8867	1,7149	0,8059	1,03
SR14	1,0573	1,1367	0,5782	1,8120	0,8069	0,8716	0,7176	1,6669	0,9569	1,3373	0,9206	1,08
SR15	1,0938	1,4109	0,5787	1,3301	0,9803	0,4940	1,6667	0,0831	1,1083	0,7058	1,2107	1,06
SR16	1,0338	0,9355	0,9658	1,3368	1,1015	0,0511	1,0906	1,0272	0,9853	1,0436	1,0645	1,06
SR17	0,9594	0,8037	0,8764	2,7446	0,4826	0,8523	1,1902	0,9569	0,9739	0,8093	1,4202	1,10
SR18	1,1452	1,5035	0,9661	1,1765	0,9744	1,5788	0,6661	1,0232	0,6305	1,0328	1,0292	1,07
SR19	0,7839	0,9507	0,9621	1,4090	0,6207	1,6541	0,6056	0,9022	1,0117	0,8725	1,4084	1,02
SR20	0,9973	1,0808	0,6325	1,7072	0,7433	1,0266	1,1143	1,3517	0,8149	0,6923	1,6585	1,07
SR21	0,7643	1,1270	0,8978	1,8138	1,1484	0,6927	1,0508	0,9265	0,9987	1,0703	1,0898	1,05
SR22	1,2577	1,2146	0,5479	2,2375	0,5990	0,9636	1,1503	1,2143	0,9435	0,7466	1,1050	1,09
SR23	0,8704	1,7757	0,5355	2,3304	0,7600	0,9115	0,8323	1,6850	0,7524	0,8580	1,4325	1,16
SR24	0,9278	0,8948	1,0328	1,7058	1,5519	0,8162	0,8653	1,1291	0,9156	0,7789	1,1645	1,07
SR26	1,2886	0,6650	2,5284	0,4481	1,2674	0,8278	1,5212	0,6854	0,8729	1,0250	1,3263	1,13
SR27	1,0889	0,9743	0,9762	1,7508	0,7002	1,1476	1,0480	1,3466	1,0194	0,8750	1,3785	1,12
SR28	0,7325	1,0951	1,0915	1,8427	0,7582	0,9706	1,0366	1,0374	0,8662	0,9406	1,1008	1,04
SR29	2,0083	0,6575	0,7820	1,4554	0,9709	1,0250	0,9906	0,7858	0,9647	1,4479	1,5096	1,15
SR30	0,7530	1,1899	0,8783	1,2557	0,9538	0,8801	0,9507	1,2133	0,8409	0,8979	1,4759	1,03
SR32	1,0415	0,9003	0,7032	1,7818	1,1913	0,8561	0,9001	1,5909	1,0360	1,0077	1,0800	1,01
SR33	0,7527	1,4469	0,8569	1,3489	0,4910	1,1037	0,8915	1,0550	1,1592	0,7451	1,4055	1,02
SR34	1,0603	0,8913	1,0332	1,1433	0,9603	1,0471	0,9734	1,0875	0,8131	0,8324	1,1498	1,00
SR35	1,2473	1,3100	0,8676	1,1190	1,2797	1,2751	0,9119	1,5445	0,3900	2,6793	0,3238	1,18
SR36	1,2639	0,9926	1,1079	1,0618	1,1755	1,0856	1,0313	0,9466	1,0341	0,8377	1,1214	1,06
SR37	0,5501	0,9992	0,9537	1,5036	0,8358	1,1706	0,7744	0,7167	0,9583	0,9867	1,0157	0,95
SR38	1,0053	0,8335	0,9672	1,5253	0,8729	0,9532	0,8911	1,2953	0,9514	0,9294	1,3568	1,05
SR39	1,1994	1,4564	0,6626	1,3675	1,2113	0,9484	0,8987	1,1857	0,8330	0,8634	0,8952	1,05
SR40	0,7087	1,2017	0,8534	0,6810	1,8441	1,0018	0,5458	1,4573	0,8132	0,9162	1,1125	1,01
SR41	1,0518	0,8338	0,9943	1,5452	0,8680	0,9951	0,9277	1,0834	1,0197	0,8539	1,0226	1,02
SR42	1,1240	1,0517	0,7278	1,1949	0,9239	1,1897	0,7425	0,5210	4,1601	0,2299	1,1581	1,18
SR43	0,9764	0,7226	0,5599	2,6838	0,5595	0,8916	1,0301	1,2894	0,8107	0,9082	1,5200	1,09
SR44	1,0778	1,6956	1,0396	0,8125	0,9214	1,1116	1,2929	0,8852	1,0654	0,8664	1,2534	1,09
SR45	0,9630	0,9412	0,9362	1,5273	1,0120	1,0958	0,9366	1,1481	0,8213	0,9264	1,1932	1,05
SR46	0,9686	1,5151	0,7616	1,2820	1,3635	1,0987	0,8454	1,1302	1,0026	0,8590	0,9676	1,07
SR47	1,3783	0,9208	0,8965	1,5569	0,8904	0,8730	1,0400	1,1970	1,5113	0,7346	1,2455	1,11
SR48	1,2273	0,9750	0,8970	1,0414	0,9472	0,8505	0,9923	0,9960	0,9481	0,9945	0,9906	0,99
SR49	0,9954	1,3059	0,4307	1,2475	0,7666	0,5363	1,2107	1,1057	0,8656	1,1235	1,0576	0,97
SR50	0,9741	0,9055	1,1773	1,4563	1,2082	0,9325	1,0774	1,0981	0,9728	1,0143	0,9919	1,07
SR51	1,1180	1,1710	0,7025	1,9049	1,0349	0,9386	0,9350	0,8439	1,1060	1,0605	0,9057	1,07
SR52	0,8541	1,3070	0,8715	1,1679	1,4045	0,8530	0,6330	1,2219	1,1505	0,9586	0,8515	1,02
SR53	0,5045	0,8208	1,2736	1,4587	1,1209	0,9421	1,1388	1,4495	1,1888	0,3786	1,1099	1,04
SR54	0,5093	0,6837	1,0690	2,0071	1,0780	0,7619	0,9222	1,6734	0,8636	1,5843	1,0565	1,11
SR55	1,0605	0,9097	0,9681	1,3847	0,9556	0,8617	1,0770	1,1838	0,9037	0,7506	1,4708	1,05
SR56	0,9762	0,9594	0,9194	1,0303	0,3472	1,1886	1,5812	0,6504	1,0491	0,7888	1,1580	0,97
SR57	0,9856	0,9447	0,9131	1,5497	0,4520	0,9928	0,9621	1,4707	0,7764	0,8437	1,3000	1,02
SR58	1,1161	1,0515	0,9081	1,9914	0,6233	1,0412	0,8612	1,2446	0,9390	0,9864	0,9741	1,07
SR59	0,9318	1,0677	0,7882	1,4159	1,0231	0,6995	1,1828	1,3646	0,8595	1,2418	1,2769	1,08
SR60	1,0108	1,1000	0,9494	1,5122	0,9627	1,1425	0,7991	1,1911	1,1384	0,7757	1,1505	1,07
SR61	0,9610	1,0340	1,0671	1,5346	1,1940	0,0164	0,9804	1,1652	0,9806	0,8239	1,4452	1,11
SR62	1,0430	0,9256	0,7716	1,6514	0,8673	0,9761	0,8002	1,1492	0,9790	0,9578	1,3266	1,04
SR63	1,3533	2,1815	0,4036	1,9697	1,1430	0,8048	1,0255	1,3956	0,7657	0,9723	1,0391	1,19
Ø	1,0114	1,0928	0,8792	1,4864	1,0185	0,9574	0,9725	1,1378	0,9908	0,9570	1,1608	1,06
Max	2,0083	2,1815	2,5284	2,7446	2,3250	1,6541	1,6667	2,0216	4,1601	2,6793	1,6585	1,19
Min	0,5045	0,6575	0,4036	0,4481	0,3472	0,1620	0,4817	0,5210	0,3900	0,2299	0,3238	0,95
SD	0,2525	0,2842	0,2810	0,4310	0,3467	0,2220	0,2260	0,2839	0,4413	0,3172	0,2193	0,05

Table 7.2.1-10: The Malmquist Productivity Index of the individual sales reps

7.2.2 Appendix B2 (CCR-Model, Version: F, CCD, CCP, F/T – Q, CI)

Sales Rep	Score	Excess F S-(1)	Excess CCD S-(2)	Excess CCP S-(3)	Excess F/T S-(4)	Shortage Q S+(1)	Shortage CI S+(2)
SR1	0,96	0	0	33,89683994	0	0	0
SR2	0,61	0	0	0	0	0	0
SR3	0,72	4,38E-03	0	43,8477181	0	0	0
SR4	1,00	0	0	0	0	0	0
SR5	0,57	0	0	0	0	0	0
SR6	1,00	0	0	0	0	0	0
SR7	0,94	0	26,68737414	17,34460191	0	0	0
SR8	0,63	0	0	40,95681655	0	0	0
SR9	0,98	0	6,704939249	71,29613744	0	0	0
SR10	0,73	0	0	0	0	0	0
SR11	0,84	7,30E-02	0	28	0,433	0	1,81E-02
SR12	0,96	0	0	0	2,24E-02	0	0
SR13	0,60	0	0	19,39402763	0	0	0
SR14	0,77	0	0	0	2,22E-02	0	0
SR15	0,95	0	0	0	0	1,893233996	0
SR16	1,00	0	0	0	0	0	0
SR17	0,71	0	0	16,48431896	0	0	0
SR18	0,71	0	0	0	0	0	0
SR19	0,76	0	0	12,61167859	4,07E-02	0	0
SR20	0,83	0	0	49,94660734	0	2,350360986	0
SR21	0,70	0	0	0	0	0	0
SR22	0,81	0	0	0	0	0	0
SR23	1,00	0,134833401	0	50,84955231	3,28E-02	0	0
SR24	0,77	0	0	2,574310657	0	0	0
SR26	0,67	0	0	35,6673035	0	0	0
SR27	0,82	0	0	32,33373285	0	0	0
SR28	0,77	0	0	0	0	0	0
SR29	0,91	0	0	26,55769991	0,167979713	0	0
SR30	0,94	0	0	25,31864508	0	0	0
SR32	1,00	0	0	0	0	0	0
SR33	0,71	0	0	18,99914436	3,79E-02	0	0
SR34	0,83	0	0	16,18119541	0	3,056080163	0
SR35	0,74	0	0	12,44271413	0	1,099974007	0
SR36	0,89	0	0	25,1859909	0	0	0
SR37	0,52	0	0	0	0	0	0
SR38	0,83	0	0	0	9,59E-02	0	0
SR39	0,72	0	0	34,08934876	0	0	0
SR40	0,81	0	0	0	0	0	0
SR41	0,71	0	0	0	0	0	0
SR42	0,60	0	0	0	0	2,964160593	0
SR43	1,00	0	0	0	0	0	0
SR44	1,00	0	0	0	0	0	0
SR45	0,81	0	0	14,59698456	0	0,375270543	0
SR46	0,90	0	0	0	0	0	0
SR47	1,00	0	0	0	0	0	0
SR48	1,00	0	0	0	0	0	0
SR49	0,78	0	0	0	0	0	0
SR50	0,94	0,069047619	52,6984127	45,07936508	0	0	1,75E-02
SR51	0,52	0	0	0	0,634339255	0	0
SR52	0,78	0	0	10,13468761	0	0	0
SR53	0,66	0	51,87649289	13,98493791	0	0	0
SR54	1,00	0	0	0	0	0	0
SR55	0,78	0	0	45,70522803	0	0,993022191	0
SR56	0,79	0	0	0	7,04E-02	0	0
SR57	0,79	3,49E-02	0	0	0	0	0
SR58	0,84	0	0	19,00542562	0	0	0
SR59	1,00	0	0	0	0	0	0
SR60	0,87	0	0	31,1826742	5,48E-02	0	0
SR61	0,81	0	0	0	0	0	0
SR62	1,00	0	0	0	0	0	0
SR63	0,68	0	0	8,518246957	0	0	0

Table 7.2.2-1: The table on the left displays the slack values for the CCR model version 1 for each sales reps

Table 7.2.2-2: The table on the left displays the virtual weights for the CCR model version 1

DMU	Score	V(1) F	V(2) CCD	V(3) CCP	V(4) F/T	U(1) Q	U(2) CI
SR1	0,96	0,53450	0,00318	0,00000	0,09570	0,04549	1,97586
SR2	0,61	0,53653	0,00348	0,00161	0,10483	0,06037	2,24169
SR3	0,72	0,00000	0,00445	0,00000	0,72211	0,02675	3,07790
SR4	1,00	0,63406	0,00206	0,00076	0,00000	0,10541	0,00000
SR5	0,57	0,70877	0,00460	0,00213	0,13848	0,07975	2,96130
SR6	1,00	1,45436	0,00000	0,00000	0,36896	0,12367	0,50961
SR7	0,94	0,70182	0,00000	0,00000	1,01341	0,08262	1,31382
SR8	0,63	0,23120	0,00366	0,00000	0,60381	0,02859	2,97596
SR9	0,98	0,72241	0,00000	0,00000	0,74446	0,07323	1,06578
SR10	0,73	0,60263	0,00223	0,00053	0,17920	0,06603	1,42354
SR11	0,84	0,00000	0,00658	0,00000	0,00000	0,13063	0,00000
SR12	0,96	0,39427	0,00308	0,00171	0,00000	0,05549	1,60177
SR13	0,60	0,26124	0,00413	0,00000	0,68227	0,03231	3,36270
SR14	0,77	0,46922	0,00295	0,00425	0,00000	0,02558	2,74411
SR15	0,95	0,06908	0,00196	0,00168	0,47878	0,00000	2,42736
SR16	1,00	0,48090	0,00286	0,00000	0,08610	0,04093	1,77772
SR17	0,71	0,60361	0,00408	0,00000	0,13086	0,06800	2,21940
SR18	0,71	0,54709	0,00355	0,00165	0,10689	0,06156	2,28580
SR19	0,76	0,58382	0,00492	0,00000	0,00000	0,08500	1,91903
SR20	0,83	0,26513	0,00248	0,00000	0,36131	0,00000	2,45111
SR21	0,70	0,07564	0,00285	0,00246	0,65314	0,01258	3,21498
SR22	0,81	0,10121	0,00240	0,00255	0,46629	0,01605	2,60775
SR23	1,00	0,00000	0,00715	0,00000	0,00000	0,09774	1,27402
SR24	0,77	0,79190	0,00197	0,00000	0,25188	0,08917	1,12011
SR26	0,67	0,50991	0,00345	0,00000	0,11055	0,05744	1,87488
SR27	0,82	0,64133	0,00434	0,00000	0,13904	0,07225	2,35812
SR28	0,77	0,24224	0,00291	0,00081	0,45618	0,02629	2,55976
SR29	0,91	0,79973	0,00414	0,00000	0,00000	0,03822	2,83472
SR30	0,94	0,16829	0,00266	0,00000	0,43953	0,02082	2,16629
SR32	1,00	0,59696	0,00222	0,00000	0,00000	0,09924	0,00000
SR33	0,71	0,85342	0,00441	0,00000	0,00000	0,04078	3,02504
SR34	0,83	0,23716	0,00274	0,00000	0,44379	0,00000	2,68974
SR35	0,74	0,36552	0,00342	0,00000	0,49812	0,00000	3,37923
SR36	0,89	0,18629	0,00295	0,00000	0,48652	0,02304	2,39791
SR37	0,52	0,09372	0,00364	0,00432	0,85908	0,01901	4,32852
SR38	0,83	0,46347	0,00291	0,00420	0,00000	0,02526	2,71052
SR39	0,72	0,19215	0,00282	0,00000	0,50854	0,02377	2,35762
SR40	0,81	0,05788	0,00225	0,00267	0,53056	0,01174	2,67326
SR41	0,71	0,19338	0,00018	0,00365	1,10601	0,00881	2,91530
SR42	0,60	0,10457	0,00274	0,00551	0,76415	0,00000	4,19295
SR43	1,00	0,00000	0,00694	0,00000	0,00000	0,09496	1,23773
SR44	1,00	0,45472	0,00249	0,00210	0,00000	0,00000	2,46563
SR45	0,81	0,25597	0,00296	0,00000	0,47899	0,00000	2,90309
SR46	0,90	0,05106	0,00192	0,00166	0,43995	0,00839	2,16677
SR47	1,00	0,00000	0,00248	0,00194	0,56946	0,00000	2,76485
SR48	1,00	0,05663	0,00213	0,00184	0,48896	0,00941	2,40681
SR49	0,78	0,06384	0,00265	0,00215	0,60949	0,01131	2,95678
SR50	1,00	0,00000	0,00000	0,00000	1,79572	0,11227	0,00000
SR51	0,52	0,32215	0,00510	0,00000	0,84136	0,03984	4,14679
SR52	0,78	0,20469	0,00300	0,00000	0,54173	0,02532	2,51153
SR53	0,66	0,31905	0,00000	0,00000	1,42855	0,05511	1,83728
SR54	1,00	2,08333	0,00000	0,00000	0,00000	0,13995	0,00000
SR55	0,78	0,29404	0,00275	0,00000	0,40071	0,00000	2,71841
SR56	0,79	0,43202	0,00271	0,00391	0,00000	0,02355	2,52658
SR57	0,79	0,00000	0,00329	0,00254	0,74204	0,01217	3,45522
SR58	0,84	0,18696	0,00296	0,00000	0,48827	0,02312	2,40650
SR59	1,00	0,00000	0,00000	0,00000	2,27273	0,09035	1,49375
SR60	0,87	0,53495	0,00451	0,00000	0,00000	0,07789	1,75839
SR61	0,81	0,41757	0,00271	0,00126	0,08159	0,04698	1,74466
SR62	1,00	0,05614	0,00000	0,00000	1,75828	0,00000	2,54653
SR63	0,68	0,34736	0,00017	0,00000	1,66705	0,06185	2,24671

DMU	Score	Benchmark	Impact	Benchmark	Impact	Benchmark	Impact	Benchmark	Impact	Benchmark	Impact
SR1	0,96	SR6	0,15	SR16	0,32	SR43	0,20	SR54	0,35		
SR2	0,61	SR4	0,41	SR6	0,31	SR32	0,13	SR43	0,12	SR54	0,32
SR3	0,72	SR32	0,46	SR43	0,23	SR62	0,34				
SR4	1,00	SR4	1,00								
SR5	0,57	SR4	0,10	SR6	0,29	SR32	0,13	SR43	0,46	SR54	0,09
SR6	1,00	SR6	1,00								
SR7	0,94	SR4	0,10	SR32	0,16	SR48	0,70				
SR8	0,63	SR16	0,61	SR32	0,00	SR43	0,29	SR62	0,29		
SR9	0,98	SR4	0,47	SR6	0,17	SR16	0,37				
SR10	0,73	SR4	0,31	SR6	0,14	SR16	0,12	SR32	0,45	SR54	0,25
SR11	0,84	SR32	0,90								
SR12	0,96	SR4	0,18	SR32	0,30	SR43	0,44	SR54	0,12		
SR13	0,60	SR16	0,47	SR32	0,06	SR43	0,20	SR62	0,39		
SR14	0,77	SR4	0,06	SR6	0,68	SR43	0,25	SR44	0,08		
SR15	0,95	SR6	0,21	SR44	0,41	SR47	0,18	SR62	0,30		
SR16	1,00	SR16	1,00								
SR17	0,71	SR16	0,60	SR32	0,09	SR43	0,30	SR54	0,09		
SR18	0,71	SR4	0,17	SR6	0,11	SR32	0,19	SR43	0,15	SR54	0,50
SR19	0,76	SR32	0,09	SR43	0,29	SR54	0,69				
SR20	0,83	SR6	0,34	SR43	0,41	SR48	0,54				
SR21	0,70	SR6	0,13	SR32	0,43	SR43	0,41	SR47	0,10	SR48	0,06
SR22	0,81	SR4	0,34	SR6	0,05	SR32	0,37	SR43	0,21	SR44	0,17
SR23	1,00	SR32	0,28	SR43	0,59						
SR24	0,77	SR4	0,06	SR16	0,41	SR32	0,23	SR54	0,47		
SR26	0,67	SR16	0,79	SR32	0,41	SR43	0,02	SR54	0,04		
SR27	0,82	SR16	0,15	SR32	0,06	SR43	0,41	SR54	0,31		
SR28	0,77	SR6	0,12	SR16	0,02	SR32	0,45	SR43	0,18	SR48	0,36
SR29	0,91	SR6	0,65	SR43	0,06	SR54	0,12				
SR30	0,94	SR16	0,07	SR32	0,11	SR43	0,13	SR62	0,80		
SR32	1,00	SR32	1,00								
SR33	0,71	SR6	0,38	SR43	0,30	SR54	0,38				
SR34	0,83	SR43	0,59	SR48	0,58	SR62	0,01				
SR35	0,74	SR6	0,27	SR43	0,47	SR48	0,31				
SR36	0,89	SR16	0,01	SR32	0,50	SR43	0,33	SR62	0,23		
SR37	0,52	SR4	0,06	SR6	0,21	SR32	0,33	SR44	0,39	SR47	0,11
SR38	0,83	SR4	0,38	SR6	0,07	SR43	0,09	SR44	0,45		
SR39	0,72	SR16	0,92	SR32	0,08	SR48	0,20	SR62	0,06		
SR40	0,81	SR4	0,35	SR6	0,10	SR32	0,23	SR44	0,41	SR47	0,05
SR41	0,71	SR4	0,34	SR6	0,47	SR47	0,38	SR48	0,02	SR59	0,02
SR42	0,60	SR4	0,05	SR6	0,13	SR44	0,67	SR47	0,17		
SR43	1,00	SR43	1,00								
SR44	1,00	SR44	1,00								
SR45	0,81	SR43	0,42	SR48	0,24	SR62	0,46				
SR46	0,90	SR6	0,49	SR43	0,23	SR44	0,14	SR47	0,18	SR48	0,23
SR47	1,00	SR47	1,00								
SR48	1,00	SR48	1,00								
SR49	0,78	SR32	0,09	SR43	0,17	SR47	0,32	SR48	0,42	SR62	0,10
SR50	0,94	SR32	0,94								
SR51	0,52	SR16	0,30	SR32	0,14	SR43	0,51	SR62	0,11		
SR52	0,78	SR16	0,47	SR32	0,03	SR48	0,05	SR62	0,57		
SR53	0,66	SR32	0,03	SR48	1,26	SR59	0,14				
SR54	1,00	SR54	1,00								
SR55	0,78	SR6	0,11	SR43	0,67	SR48	0,47				
SR56	0,79	SR4	0,08	SR6	0,39	SR43	0,12	SR44	0,52		
SR57	0,79	SR32	0,27	SR43	0,40	SR47	0,22	SR62	0,06		
SR58	0,84	SR16	0,21	SR32	0,22	SR43	0,15	SR62	0,53		
SR59	1,00	SR59	1,00								
SR60	0,87	SR32	0,18	SR43	0,22	SR54	0,60				
SR61	0,81	SR4	0,43	SR6	0,19	SR32	0,14	SR43	0,14	SR54	0,35
SR62	1,00	SR62	1,00								
SR63	0,68	SR32	0,19	SR48	0,53	SR59	0,18	SR62	0,26		

Table 7.2.2-3: The table on the left displays the individual benchmark partners for inefficient sales reps for the CCR model version 1 (remember: Returns to Scale = Constant (0 =< Sum of Lambda < Infinity))

	F		CCD		CCP		F/T		Q		CI	
Sales Rep	Status Quo	Target	Status Quo	Target	Status Quo	Target	Status Quo	Target	Status Quo	Target	Status Quo	Target
SR1	0,62	0,62	200	200	120	86	0,83	0,83	6,79	7,10	0,35	0,37
SR2	0,84	0,84	273	273	84	84	1,00	1,00	6,20	10,18	0,28	0,46
SR3	0,93	0,93	200	200	140	96	0,68	0,68	5,78	7,97	0,27	0,38
SR4	0,75	0,75	240	240	40	40	0,72	0,72	9,49	9,49	0,36	0,36
SR5	0,77	0,77	200	200	80	80	0,85	0,85	4,25	7,46	0,22	0,39
SR6	0,51	0,51	228	228	76	76	0,70	0,70	6,48	6,48	0,39	0,39
SR7	0,65	0,65	240	213	100	83	0,60	0,60	6,71	7,15	0,34	0,36
SR8	0,90	0,90	240	240	160	119	0,83	0,83	5,12	8,13	0,29	0,46
SR9	0,68	0,68	240	233	140	69	0,71	0,71	8,26	8,43	0,37	0,38
SR10	0,92	0,92	270	270	90	90	0,92	0,92	8,09	11,09	0,33	0,45
SR11	0,91	0,84	180	180	100	72	1,00	0,57	7,66	9,07	0,25	0,31
SR12	0,84	0,84	190	190	76	76	0,85	0,83	7,79	8,15	0,35	0,37
SR13	0,87	0,87	228	228	133	114	0,74	0,74	4,56	7,64	0,25	0,42
SR14	0,67	0,67	220	220	80	80	0,84	0,82	5,25	6,84	0,32	0,41
SR15	0,90	0,90	228	228	95	95	0,80	0,80	4,25	6,36	0,41	0,43
SR16	0,65	0,65	220	220	100	100	0,68	0,68	7,73	7,73	0,38	0,38
SR17	0,76	0,76	209	209	114	98	0,81	0,81	5,54	7,85	0,28	0,40
SR18	0,72	0,72	220	220	80	80	0,92	0,92	6,15	8,64	0,27	0,38
SR19	0,65	0,65	190	190	95	82	1,00	0,96	5,68	7,46	0,27	0,35
SR20	0,85	0,85	260	260	160	110	0,94	0,94	4,82	8,18	0,41	0,49
SR21	0,93	0,93	210	210	90	90	0,82	0,82	5,96	8,49	0,29	0,41
SR22	0,95	0,95	228	228	76	76	0,86	0,86	7,60	9,41	0,34	0,42
SR23	0,88	0,75	140	140	120	69	0,73	0,70	6,17	6,17	0,31	0,31
SR24	0,75	0,75	240	240	100	97	0,91	0,91	7,26	9,41	0,31	0,41
SR26	0,93	0,93	266	266	152	116	0,85	0,85	7,16	10,63	0,31	0,47
SR27	0,64	0,64	162	162	108	76	0,79	0,79	5,16	6,31	0,27	0,33
SR28	0,86	0,86	228	228	95	95	0,76	0,76	6,83	8,84	0,32	0,41
SR29	0,44	0,44	180	180	90	63	0,79	0,62	4,95	5,42	0,29	0,31
SR30	0,97	0,97	231	231	147	122	0,66	0,66	6,65	7,11	0,40	0,42
SR32	0,93	0,93	200	200	80	80	0,63	0,63	10,08	10,08	0,35	0,35
SR33	0,62	0,62	200	200	100	81	0,92	0,88	4,84	6,84	0,27	0,37
SR34	0,86	0,86	220	220	120	104	0,89	0,89	3,56	7,34	0,37	0,45
SR35	0,72	0,72	200	200	100	88	0,80	0,80	4,03	6,53	0,30	0,40
SR36	0,95	0,95	200	200	120	95	0,74	0,74	7,43	8,37	0,35	0,39
SR37	0,89	0,89	220	220	80	80	0,82	0,82	4,06	7,86	0,21	0,41
SR38	0,79	0,79	200	200	60	60	0,92	0,82	5,77	6,93	0,32	0,38
SR39	0,86	0,86	280	280	160	126	0,84	0,84	7,02	9,70	0,35	0,49
SR40	0,92	0,92	234	234	72	72	0,87	0,87	7,00	8,63	0,34	0,42
SR41	0,86	0,86	280	280	80	80	0,81	0,81	6,12	8,61	0,32	0,46
SR42	0,84	0,84	198	198	72	72	0,85	0,85	1,69	5,79	0,24	0,40
SR43	0,83	0,83	144	144	80	80	0,89	0,89	5,75	5,75	0,37	0,37
SR44	0,88	0,88	180	180	72	72	0,94	0,94	5,33	5,33	0,41	0,41
SR45	0,91	0,91	216	216	126	111	0,77	0,77	5,13	6,75	0,34	0,43
SR46	0,86	0,86	260	260	100	100	0,92	0,92	6,94	7,73	0,43	0,48
SR47	0,88	0,88	216	216	72	72	0,57	0,57	5,50	5,50	0,36	0,36
SR48	0,62	0,62	228	228	95	95	0,62	0,62	6,68	6,68	0,39	0,39
SR49	0,85	0,85	228	228	95	95	0,70	0,70	5,42	6,99	0,32	0,41
SR50	0,94	0,87	240	187	120	75	0,59	0,59	8,91	9,44	0,29	0,33
SR51	0,84	0,84	190	190	95	94	0,80	0,80	3,80	7,26	0,20	0,39
SR52	0,88	0,88	247	247	133	123	0,68	0,68	5,97	7,70	0,34	0,44
SR53	0,93	0,93	378	326	147	133	0,86	0,86	6,23	9,50	0,36	0,55
SR54	0,48	0,48	190	190	76	76	0,94	0,94	7,15	7,15	0,32	0,32
SR55	0,90	0,90	228	228	152	106	0,96	0,96	5,23	7,68	0,37	0,47
SR56	0,82	0,82	220	220	80	80	1,00	0,93	5,37	6,79	0,35	0,44
SR57	0,86	0,83	171	171	76	76	0,68	0,68	5,20	6,55	0,27	0,34
SR58	0,94	0,94	228	228	133	114	0,70	0,70	6,58	7,84	0,35	0,42
SR59	0,88	0,88	240	240	80	80	0,44	0,44	5,72	5,72	0,32	0,32
SR60	0,63	0,63	180	180	108	77	0,92	0,87	6,35	7,29	0,29	0,33
SR61	0,83	0,83	260	260	80	80	0,98	0,98	8,11	9,99	0,35	0,44
SR62	0,90	0,90	220	220	120	120	0,54	0,54	5,95	5,95	0,39	0,39
SR63	0,90	0,90	260	260	120	111	0,67	0,67	5,47	8,06	0,29	0,43

Table 7.2.2-4: The table on the left displays the status quo value for q4 2006 and the optimized target values for the CCR model version 1

7.2.3 Appendix B3 (BCC-Model, Version: F, CCD, CCP, F/T – Q, CI)

DMU	Score	Excess F S-(1)	Excess CCD S-(2)	Excess CCP S-(3)	Excess F/T S-(4)	Shortage Q S+(1)	Shortage CI S+(2)
SR1	0,96	0	0	33	0,04392	0	0
SR2	0,72	0	35	10	0,221509	0	0
SR3	0,74	2,05E-02	0	51	0	0	0
SR4	1,00	0	0	0	0	0	0
SR5	0,59	0	0	0	0,071471	0	0
SR6	1,00	0	0	0	0	0	0
SR7	1,00	0	0	0	0	0	0
SR8	0,70	0,021572	0	64	0	0	0
SR9	0,99	0	11	67	0,011942	0	0
SR10	0,88	0,009178	54	5	0,210548	0	0
SR11	0,87	0,00E+00	0	7	0,334468	0	5,06E-02
SR12	0,97	0	0	0	9,76E-02	0	0
SR13	0,63	0	0	33	0	0	0
SR14	0,80	0	0	0	6,04E-02	0	0
SR15	1,00	0	0	0	0	0	0
SR16	1,00	0	0	0	0	0	0
SR17	0,73	0	0	24	0,071575	0	0
SR18	0,73	0	0	0	0,226422	0	0
SR19	0,77	0	0	11	1,77E-01	0	0
SR20	0,94	0	1	61	0,026286	1,814493418	0
SR21	0,75	0,031414	0	7	0,03216	0	0
SR22	0,88	0,090292	0	0	0,095406	0	0
SR23	1,00	9,94E-06	0	0	0,00E+00	0	0
SR24	0,83	0	0	38	0,162623	0	0
SR26	0,82	0,029294	41	64	0,09864	0	0
SR27	0,93	0	0	5	0,025183	0	0,01352151
SR28	0,82	0	0	3	0	0	0
SR29	1,00	0	0	0	9,97E-06	0	0
SR30	0,99	0,078301	2	37	0	0	0
SR32	1,00	0	0	0	0	0	0
SR33	0,71	0	0	16	1,43E-01	0	0
SR34	0,89	0	0	32	0	2,14936437	0
SR35	0,75	0	0	21	0	0,608490842	0
SR36	0,92	0,042803	0	38	0	0	0
SR37	0,54	0,0318	0	0	0	0	0
SR38	0,84	0	0	0	1,03E-01	0,491655714	0
SR39	0,87	0	37	73	0,015241	0	0
SR40	0,87	0,088028	0	0	0,054498	0	0
SR41	0,80	0,087063	32	0	0	0	0
SR42	0,60	0,081135	0	0	0	3,039203659	0
SR43	1,00	0	0	0	0	0	0
SR44	1,00	0	0	0	0	0	0
SR45	0,85	0,02605	0	28	0	0	0
SR46	1,00	0	0	0	0	0	0
SR47	1,00	0	0	0	0	0	0
SR48	1,00	0	0	0	0	0	0
SR49	0,80	0,121316	0	0	0	0	0
SR50	0,97	0,020534	32	40	0	0	4,33E-02
SR51	0,53	0	0	14	0	0	0
SR52	0,85	0	18	27	0	0	0
SR53	0,85	0,058181	128	49	0	0	0
SR54	1,00	0	0	0	0	0	0
SR55	0,87	0,032	0	63	0,032	0,277251621	0
SR56	0,84	0	1	0	1,12E-01	0	0
SR57	1,00	0,00E+00	0	0	0	0	0
SR58	0,89	0,046054	0	31	0	0	0
SR59	1,00	0	0	0	0	0	0
SR60	0,88	0	0	27	4,89E-02	0	0
SR61	0,93	0	22	10	0,21196	0	0
SR62	1,00	0	0	0	0	0	0
SR63	0,75	0,003502	34	16	0	0	0

Table 7.2.3-1: The table on the left displays the slack values for the BCC model version 1 for each sales reps

DMU	Score	V(1) F	V(2) CCD	V(3) CCP	V(4) F/T	U(1) Q	U(2) CI	Free Variable
SR1	0,95966	0,47589	0,00273	0,00000	0,00000	0,04345	2,0153	0,20094808
SR2	0,72064	0,07618	0,00000	0,00000	0,00000	0,06196	2,2064	1,32366756
SR3	0,73523	0,00000	0,00256	0,00000	0,31264	0,02693	3,0742	0,63574568
SR4	1,00000	0,63406	0,00206	0,00076	0,00000	0,10541	0	0
SR5	0,58584	0,33781	0,00277	0,00122	0,00000	0,05751	3,3847	0,79543114
SR6	1,00000	1,45436	0,00000	0,00000	0,36896	0,12367	0,5096	0
SR7	1,00000	1,54596	0,00000	0,00000	2,12762	0,14766	0,0251	-1,28144912
SR8	0,69534	0,00000	0,00171	0,00000	0,22282	0,02814	2,9841	0,84310225
SR9	0,98920	0,32976	0,00000	0,00000	0,00000	0,04350	1,7287	0,78667587
SR10	0,87798	0,00000	0,00000	0,00000	0,00000	0,04983	1,8245	1,13897303
SR11	0,87429	0,67412	0,00795	0,00000	0,00000	0,13063	0	-0,90127429
SR12	0,97027	0,20504	0,00168	0,00074	0,00000	0,03491	2,0544	0,48279712
SR13	0,63341	0,02399	0,00194	0,00000	0,25351	0,03194	3,3694	0,92814958
SR14	0,79591	0,19318	0,00145	0,00079	0,00000	0,03710	2,5523	0,74492954
SR15	1,00000	0,00000	0,00053	0,00136	0,29396	0,00000	2,4274	0,51492633
SR16	1,00000	0,48090	0,00286	0,00000	0,08610	0,04093	1,7777	0
SR17	0,73008	0,13791	0,00187	0,00000	0,00000	0,04185	2,7345	0,87314448
SR18	0,72982	0,26519	0,00217	0,00096	0,00000	0,04515	2,657	0,62442814
SR19	0,77182	0,52643	0,00354	0,00000	0,00000	0,06732	2,2919	0,28170458
SR20	0,94150	0,31776	0,00000	0,00000	0,00000	0,00000	2,4511	0,79203862
SR21	0,74502	0,00000	0,00176	0,00000	0,00000	0,03910	2,6659	0,97276949
SR22	0,88007	0,00000	0,00112	0,00103	0,00000	0,03291	2,2274	0,80392097
SR23	1,00000	0,00000	0,00718	0,00000	0,00000	0,09813	1,2662	-0,00533066
SR24	0,83422	0,31633	0,00000	0,00000	0,00000	0,04771	2,0759	0,96148175
SR26	0,81626	0,00000	0,00000	0,00000	0,00000	0,05359	1,9625	1,22510139
SR27	0,93394	3,23263	0,02966	0,00000	0,00000	0,19367	0	-5,80262119
SR28	0,81972	0,01848	0,00149	0,00000	0,19529	0,02460	2,5957	0,71500997
SR29	1,00000	1,24793	0,00569	0,00000	0,00000	0,00054	3,4862	-0,5733563
SR30	0,99409	0,00000	0,00000	0,00000	0,29892	0,02814	2,0437	0,80866425
SR32	1,00000	0,59696	0,00222	0,00000	0,00000	0,09924	0	0
SR33	0,71499	0,63874	0,00366	0,00000	0,00000	0,05832	2,705	0,26971187
SR34	0,89219	0,11882	0,00106	0,00000	0,19817	0,00000	2,6897	0,60997638
SR35	0,75112	0,26940	0,00276	0,00000	0,36594	0,00000	3,3792	0,29320595
SR36	0,91906	0,00000	0,00138	0,00000	0,17962	0,02268	2,4056	0,67965354
SR37	0,53923	0,00000	0,00153	0,00192	0,45380	0,02923	4,1337	0,99127319
SR38	0,84207	0,81432	0,00440	0,00953	0,00000	0,00000	3,1735	-0,90813915
SR39	0,87434	0,06272	0,00000	0,00000	0,00000	0,05101	1,8165	1,08978192
SR40	0,87369	0,00000	0,00112	0,00103	0,00000	0,03307	2,2385	0,80794359
SR41	0,80343	0,00000	0,00000	0,00186	0,41565	0,00930	2,9061	0,75893209
SR42	0,59935	0,00000	0,00137	0,00428	0,63082	0,00000	4,1929	0,55243149
SR43	1,00000	0,00000	0,00694	0,00000	0,00000	0,09496	1,2377	0
SR44	1,00000	0,45472	0,00249	0,00210	0,00000	0,00000	2,4656	0
SR45	0,84723	0,00000	0,00146	0,00000	0,19006	0,02400	2,5454	0,71914909
SR46	1,00000	0,00000	0,00066	0,00114	0,23974	0,01157	2,116	0,4929292
SR47	1,00000	0,00000	0,00248	0,00194	0,56946	0,00000	2,7649	0
SR48	1,00000	0,05663	0,00213	0,00184	0,48896	0,00941	2,4068	0
SR49	0,79907	0,00000	0,00111	0,00112	0,30416	0,02009	2,807	0,67910834
SR50	0,97234	0,00000	0,00000	0,00000	2,57145	0,11227	0	-0,48871524
SR51	0,53479	0,09909	0,00335	0,00000	0,41503	0,03781	4,1846	0,81879252
SR52	0,84895	0,03913	0,00000	0,00000	0,35243	0,03309	2,3744	0,9038432
SR53	0,84990	0,00000	0,00000	0,00000	0,33002	0,03107	2,2564	0,89279384
SR54	1,00000	2,08333	0,00000	0,00000	0,00000	0,13995	0	0
SR55	0,86964	0,00000	0,00000	0,00099	0,00000	0,00000	2,7184	0,92483952
SR56	0,84228	0,15366	0,00000	0,00320	0,00000	0,00225	2,8573	0,80489633
SR57	1,00000	0,00000	0,01635	0,01107	3,46810	0,01693	3,3639	-4,99446556
SR58	0,89043	0,00000	0,00138	0,00000	0,18020	0,02276	2,4134	0,68184216
SR59	1,00000	0,00000	0,00000	0,00000	2,27273	0,09035	1,4937	0
SR60	0,87603	0,66394	0,00771	0,00000	0,00000	0,11871	0,856	-0,66541859
SR61	0,92670	0,05927	0,00000	0,00000	0,00000	0,04821	1,7167	1,02990305
SR62	1,00000	0,05614	0,00000	0,00000	1,75828	0,00000	2,5465	0
SR63	0,74927	0,00000	0,00000	0,00000	0,39541	0,03722	2,7035	1,06970947

Table 7.2.3-2: The table on the left displays the virtual weights for the BCC model version 1

DMU	Score	Benchmark	Impact	Benchmark	Impact	Benchmark	Impact	Benchmark	Impact	Benchmark	Impact
SR1	0,96	SR6	0,13	SR16	0,44	SR43	0,18	SR54	0,26		
SR2	0,72	SR4	0,34	SR32	0,25	SR46	0,41				
SR3	0,74	SR32	0,50	SR43	0,01	SR44	0,23	SR62	0,26		
SR4	1,00	SR4	1,00								
SR5	0,59	SR4	0,14	SR16	0,38	SR32	0,08	SR43	0,15	SR44	0,25
SR6	1,00	SR6	1,00								
SR7	1,00	SR7	1,00								
SR8	0,70	SR32	0,19	SR44	0,06	SR46	0,66	SR62	0,09		
SR9	0,99	SR4	0,41	SR6	0,08	SR16	0,51				
SR10	0,88	SR32	0,73	SR46	0,27						
SR11	0,87	SR23	0,33	SR32	0,66	SR54	0,01				
SR12	0,97	SR4	0,14	SR16	0,11	SR32	0,37	SR43	0,28	SR44	0,10
SR13	0,63	SR16	0,08	SR32	0,19	SR44	0,08	SR46	0,37	SR62	0,28
SR14	0,80	SR4	0,05	SR6	0,45	SR16	0,15	SR44	0,23	SR46	0,12
SR15	1,00	SR15	1,00								
SR16	1,00	SR16	1,00								
SR17	0,73	SR16	0,56	SR32	0,18	SR44	0,22	SR46	0,04		
SR18	0,73	SR4	0,28	SR16	0,56	SR32	0,12	SR43	0,04	SR44	0,00
SR19	0,77	SR16	0,27	SR32	0,12	SR43	0,20	SR54	0,41		
SR20	0,94	SR6	0,03	SR46	0,97						
SR21	0,75	SR32	0,47	SR44	0,27	SR46	0,26				
SR22	0,88	SR4	0,25	SR32	0,37	SR44	0,06	SR46	0,32		
SR23	1,00	SR23	1,00								
SR24	0,83	SR4	0,63	SR16	0,19	SR46	0,18				
SR26	0,82	SR32	0,58	SR46	0,42						
SR27	0,93	SR23	0,45	SR29	0,53	SR54	0,01				
SR28	0,82	SR16	0,14	SR32	0,42	SR44	0,01	SR46	0,42	SR62	0,01
SR29	1,00	SR29	1,00								
SR30	0,99	SR32	0,11	SR46	0,29	SR62	0,60				
SR32	1,00	SR32	1,00								
SR33	0,71	SR6	0,32	SR16	0,29	SR43	0,23	SR54	0,16		
SR34	0,89	SR44	0,45	SR46	0,44	SR48	0,05	SR62	0,06		
SR35	0,75	SR6	0,26	SR43	0,09	SR44	0,42	SR48	0,23		
SR36	0,92	SR32	0,55	SR44	0,30	SR46	0,08	SR62	0,07		
SR37	0,54	SR4	0,12	SR32	0,23	SR44	0,28	SR46	0,32	SR48	0,04
SR38	0,84	SR4	0,45	SR6	0,05	SR43	0,26	SR44	0,25		
SR39	0,87	SR4	0,15	SR32	0,23	SR46	0,63				
SR40	0,87	SR4	0,36	SR32	0,12	SR44	0,14	SR46	0,38		
SR41	0,80	SR4	0,29	SR6	0,08	SR46	0,51	SR48	0,11		
SR42	0,60	SR4	0,04	SR6	0,31	SR44	0,63	SR47	0,02		
SR43	1,00	SR43	1,00								
SR44	1,00	SR44	1,00								
SR45	0,85	SR32	0,02	SR44	0,34	SR46	0,25	SR62	0,40		
SR46	1,00	SR46	1,00								
SR47	1,00	SR47	1,00								
SR48	1,00	SR48	1,00								
SR49	0,80	SR32	0,06	SR44	0,08	SR46	0,20	SR48	0,58	SR62	0,07
SR50	0,97	SR32	0,79	SR59	0,21						
SR51	0,53	SR16	0,21	SR32	0,26	SR43	0,10	SR44	0,43	SR62	0,00
SR52	0,85	SR16	0,05	SR32	0,16	SR46	0,31	SR62	0,47		
SR53	0,85	SR32	0,14	SR46	0,81	SR62	0,05				
SR54	1,00	SR54	1,00								
SR55	0,87	SR44	0,40	SR46	0,60						
SR56	0,84	SR4	0,08	SR6	0,11	SR44	0,44	SR46	0,36		
SR57	1,00	SR57	1,00								
SR58	0,89	SR32	0,27	SR44	0,01	SR46	0,35	SR62	0,38		
SR59	1,00	SR59	1,00								
SR60	0,88	SR23	0,09	SR32	0,14	SR43	0,15	SR54	0,62		
SR61	0,93	SR4	0,42	SR32	0,23	SR46	0,35				
SR62	1,00	SR62	1,00								
SR63	0,75	SR32	0,26	SR46	0,28	SR62	0,46				

Table 7.2.3-3: The table on the left displays the individual benchmark partners for inefficient sales reps for the CCR model version 1 (remember: Returns to Scale = Constant (0 =< Sum of Lambda < Infinity))

Table 7.2.3-4: The table on the left displays the status quo value for q4 2006 and the optimized target values for the BCC model version 1

Sales Rep	F Status Quo	F Target	CCD Status Quo	CCD Target	CCP Status Quo	CCP Target	F/T Status Quo	F/T Target	Q Status Quo	Q Target	CI Status Quo	CI Target
SR1	0,62	0,62	200	200	120	87	0,83	0,79	6,7855055	7,0707	0,35	0,36
SR2	0,84	0,84	273	238	84	74	1,00	0,78	6,2000055	8,6035	0,28	0,39
SR3	0,93	0,91	200	200	140	89	0,68	0,68	5,7785054	7,8594	0,27	0,37
SR4	0,75	0,75	240	240	40	40	0,72	0,72	9,487009	9,487	0,36	0,36
SR5	0,77	0,77	200	200	80	80	0,85	0,78	4,2500042	7,2546	0,22	0,38
SR6	0,51	0,51	228	228	76	76	0,70	0,70	6,4820059	6,482	0,39	0,39
SR7	0,65	0,65	240	240	100	100	0,60	0,60	6,7145064	6,7145	0,34	0,34
SR8	0,90	0,88	240	240	160	96	0,83	0,83	5,1220046	7,3661	0,29	0,41
SR9	0,68	0,68	240	229	140	73	0,71	0,70	8,2620078	8,3522	0,37	0,37
SR10	0,92	0,91	270	216	90	85	0,92	0,71	8,0935074	9,2183	0,33	0,37
SR11	0,91	0,91	180	180	100	93	1,00	0,67	7,6550068	8,7557	0,25	0,34
SR12	0,84	0,84	190	190	76	76	0,85	0,75	7,7930074	8,0318	0,35	0,37
SR13	0,87	0,87	228	228	133	100	0,74	0,74	4,561504	7,2015	0,25	0,40
SR14	0,67	0,67	220	220	80	80	0,84	0,78	5,2520048	6,5988	0,32	0,40
SR15	0,90	0,90	228	228	95	95	0,80	0,80	4,2470037	4,247	0,41	0,41
SR16	0,65	0,65	220	220	100	100	0,68	0,68	7,7270071	7,727	0,38	0,38
SR17	0,76	0,76	209	209	114	90	0,81	0,74	5,5360049	7,5828	0,28	0,38
SR18	0,72	0,72	220	220	80	80	0,92	0,69	6,1500052	8,4267	0,27	0,37
SR19	0,65	0,65	190	190	95	84	1,00	0,82	5,6810053	7,3605	0,27	0,35
SR20	0,85	0,85	260	259	160	99	0,94	0,91	4,8170046	6,9308	0,41	0,43
SR21	0,93	0,90	210	210	90	83	0,82	0,79	5,9555056	7,9938	0,29	0,39
SR22	0,95	0,86	228	228	76	76	0,86	0,76	7,5965068	8,6317	0,34	0,38
SR23	0,88	0,88	140	140	120	120	0,73	0,73	6,1655053	6,1655	0,31	0,31
SR24	0,75	0,75	240	240	100	62	0,91	0,75	7,2585069	8,701	0,31	0,38
SR26	0,93	0,90	266	225	152	88	0,85	0,75	7,1550068	8,7656	0,31	0,38
SR27	0,64	0,64	162	162	108	103	0,79	0,76	5,1635046	5,5287	0,27	0,30
SR28	0,86	0,86	228	228	95	92	0,76	0,76	6,8310065	8,3334	0,32	0,39
SR29	0,44	0,44	180	180	90	90	0,79	0,79	4,9465044	4,9465	0,29	0,29
SR30	0,97	0,89	231	229	147	110	0,66	0,66	6,6530063	6,6926	0,40	0,40
SR32	0,93	0,93	200	200	80	80	0,63	0,63	10,076509	10,077	0,35	0,35
SR33	0,62	0,62	200	200	100	84	0,92	0,78	4,8415043	6,7714	0,27	0,37
SR34	0,86	0,86	220	220	120	88	0,89	0,89	3,5615032	6,1413	0,37	0,42
SR35	0,72	0,72	200	200	100	79	0,80	0,80	4,0305035	5,9745	0,30	0,39
SR36	0,95	0,91	200	200	120	82	0,74	0,74	7,4320066	8,0865	0,35	0,38
SR37	0,89	0,86	220	220	80	80	0,82	0,82	4,0625035	7,5339	0,21	0,40
SR38	0,79	0,79	200	200	60	60	0,92	0,82	5,7740053	7,3486	0,32	0,37
SR39	0,86	0,86	280	243	160	87	0,84	0,82	7,0195065	8,0283	0,35	0,40
SR40	0,92	0,83	234	234	72	72	0,87	0,82	6,9975066	8,0091	0,34	0,39
SR41	0,86	0,77	280	248	80	80	0,81	0,81	6,1230058	7,6211	0,32	0,40
SR42	0,84	0,76	198	198	72	72	0,85	0,85	1,6870016	5,8539	0,24	0,40
SR43	0,83	0,83	144	144	80	80	0,89	0,89	5,7500048	5,75	0,37	0,37
SR44	0,88	0,88	180	180	72	72	0,94	0,94	5,3250049	5,325	0,41	0,41
SR45	0,91	0,88	216	216	126	98	0,77	0,77	5,1335048	6,0592	0,34	0,41
SR46	0,86	0,86	260	260	100	100	0,92	0,92	6,9440063	6,944	0,43	0,43
SR47	0,88	0,88	216	216	72	72	0,57	0,57	5,499755	5,4998	0,36	0,36
SR48	0,62	0,62	228	228	95	95	0,62	0,62	6,6800054	6,68	0,39	0,39
SR49	0,85	0,73	228	228	95	95	0,70	0,70	5,4175051	6,7797	0,32	0,40
SR50	0,94	0,92	240	208	120	80	0,59	0,59	8,907008	9,1604	0,29	0,34
SR51	0,84	0,84	190	190	95	81	0,80	0,80	3,7955034	7,0971	0,20	0,38
SR52	0,88	0,88	247	229	133	106	0,68	0,68	5,9680052	7,0299	0,34	0,40
SR53	0,93	0,87	378	250	147	98	0,86	0,86	6,2295057	7,3297	0,36	0,42
SR54	0,48	0,48	190	190	76	76	0,94	0,94	7,1145065	7,1455	0,32	0,32
SR55	0,90	0,87	228	228	152	89	0,96	0,93	5,2345038	6,2964	0,37	0,42
SR56	0,82	0,82	220	219	80	80	1,00	0,89	5,3685045	6,3737	0,35	0,41
SR57	0,86	0,86	171	171	76	76	0,68	0,68	5,198505	5,1985	0,27	0,27
SR58	0,94	0,89	228	228	133	102	0,70	0,70	6,5775063	7,3869	0,35	0,40
SR59	0,88	0,88	240	240	80	80	0,44	0,44	5,724755	5,7248	0,32	0,32
SR60	0,63	0,63	180	180	108	81	0,92	0,87	6,3520058	7,2509	0,29	0,33
SR61	0,83	0,83	260	238	80	70	0,98	0,77	8,1055078	8,7466	0,35	0,38
SR62	0,90	0,90	220	220	120	120	0,54	0,54	5,9530056	5,953	0,39	0,39
SR63	0,90	0,90	260	226	120	104	0,67	0,67	5,4660053	7,2951	0,29	0,39

7.2.4 Appendix B4 (input orientated SBM model with CRS)

This section was introduced into the thesis to demonstrate the procedure using the Mann Whitney U Test to detect differences between the quartiles regarding the shadow prices and to present the conclusions that can be drawn from the results.

DMU	(I)Input 1	(I)Input 2	(O)Output 1	DMU	(I)Input 1	(I)Input 2	(O)Output 1
1	3.695701885	7.084241978	1	51	3.76632253	9.170677868	1
2	3.303659028	9.533818945	1	52	3.393511	5.002840004	1
3	2.034736611	5.903786235	1	53	2.86001984	8.767057906	1
4	3.77485718	6.783153172	1	54	3.72291486	9.044173805	1
5	3.479431381	7.361434383	1	55	2.9149782	9.654205544	1
6	3.860071695	4.832224188	1	56	3.6385691	5.557286264	1
7	3.754325676	5.877918872	1	57	2.87308157	3.98954273	1
8	2.563823266	5.894989902	1	58	2.94351468	3.941204579	1
9	3.688900527	6.608099639	1	59	3.02373834	8.449808013	1
10	2.893551836	1.196316302	1	60	2.10824544	5.720021697	1
11	3.677061586	4.266184495	1	61	3.45372236	7.736435963	1
12	3.358058319	8.64113093	1	62	3.15672146	8.100867986	1
13	2.354641729	3.08617029	1	63	3.3560801	1.436450776	1
14	3.403276595	1.240360964	1	64	3.61072685	7.320329095	1
15	3.043986498	3.476668606	1	65	3.40021354	8.736862015	1
16	2.583199954	1.609824906	1	66	3.18476976	9.994848194	1
17	3.959165497	6.385541602	1	67	2.86885309	6.563955955	1
18	3.548225628	3.516058002	1	68	2.90483734	9.066511548	1
19	2.468155825	4.617516711	1	69	2.45167862	3.933167432	1
20	3.52528852	7.339474592	1	70	2.89251553	8.130878616	1
21	3.879768374	9.376051332	1	71	2.17886779	9.667809221	1
22	3.407352429	9.201167807	1	72	3.99520428	7.31430991	1
23	3.708955772	5.995193804	1	73	3.035269	5.709298817	1
24	2.334273594	6.832918073	1	74	2.6894292	1.682033751	1
25	2.830780493	5.789131627	1	75	3.73167976	3.724132638	1
26	3.926857492	4.160192795	1	76	2.39840944	1.525424412	1
27	3.324765266	2.604089253	1	77	2.90509536	8.316108476	1
28	2.583780568	6.20894602	1	78	3.59316673	9.277438848	1
29	3.815885822	9.706655943	1	79	3.70025102	1.662696539	1
30	3.214618164	1.421372351	1	80	2.29831499	6.869999192	1
31	2.573342297	3.172358281	1	81	2.224	2.23	1
32	2.341902834	3.374410917	1	82	3.98828326	6.764621268	1
33	2.576807994	6.678916238	1	83	2.9931989	5.341875585	1
34	2.209830625	6.965925852	1	84	2.58004385	5.017358402	1
35	3.554066506	3.424062239	1	85	2.09426691	6.29429735	1
36	2.746537139	4.729344807	1	86	2.12900958	6.466563477	1
37	3.303478171	3.909887337	1	87	3.58853314	4.314615513	1
38	2.203166124	7.569916265	1	88	3.08969632	2.730271181	1
39	2.969445621	3.397055315	1	89	3.4113461	5.306023035	1
40	2.799764299	6.972284368	1	90	3.15551441	1.177300914	1
41	2.485580868	6.071236686	1	91	3.25611002	4.250794049	1
42	2.225483235	4.044728856	1	92	3.32678149	3.570738365	1
43	2.841953722	3.673657261	1	93	2.62708367	9.261816263	1
44	3.489240799	3.988325907	1	94	2.55083186	1.642584233	1
45	3.42865811	7.439357274	1	95	3.23945794	5.797313599	1
46	3.52774729	7.333412801	1	96	3.23970355	2.568278125	1
47	3.215215993	7.31211407	1	97	3.00154042	5.028738617	1
48	2.562566406	2.185441496	1	98	3.54633949	9.755563	1
49	3.630803381	5.86784233	1	99	2.54333548	9.987663472	1
50	3.699567694	7.004904893	1	100	3.76353599	7.927315183	1

Table 7.2.4-1: Data set with big variations in input 1 and input 2.

Table 7.2.4-2 and Table 7.2.4-4 check for differences between the quartiles regarding the shadow prices for the respective input dimensions. The higher the mean rank of a quartile compared to another quartile is, the higher are the shadow prices. This in turn means that the leverage effect on efficiency indicated by the shadow prices of a quartile is significantly higher than in the other quartiles. Hence, a quartile with higher shadow prices uses inputs more intense with respect to efficiency. If there are no differences between the shadow prices of quartiles, each quartile uses the inputs of such a dimension in same intensity with respect to efficiency.

To simulate such occurrences the author created Table 7.2.4-1 and Table 7.2.4-3. The first table was created with big differences in the input 1 and 2 and the latter table was created with big differences in input 1 and very small differences in input 2.

The results of Table 7.2.4-2 show that there are big differences within the shadow prices between the quartiles for the case of big variations in input 1 and 2. Hence, higher efficiency scores are accompanied by higher shadow prices. Thus, the more efficient a unit is the more intensive it is in the use of the inputs one and two.

For Table 7.2.4-4 this does not hold. The shadow prices for input 1 are significantly different between the quartiles. For input 2 no significant difference is detected. Therefore, all quartiles use input 2 more or less in the same intensity. This means that input 2 is the same importance for efficiency across the quartiles.

Dimension	Quartils	Mean Rank	z-value	double side p-value
	1 Quartile	51.1	-3.68	0.0002
	2+3 Quartile	31.4		
Input 1	1 Quartile	37.3	5.7	<.0001
	4Quartile	13		
	2+3 Quartile	7	5.48	<.0001
	4Quartile	18.5		
	1 Quartile	54.2	4.55	<.0001
	2+3 Quartile	29.9		
Input 2	1 Quartile	37	5.57	<.0001
	4Quartile	14		
	2+3 Quartile	45.2	-4.06	<.0001
	4Quartile	23.5		

Table 7.2.4-2: Results of the MWU-Test with big variations in input 2.

DMU	(I)Input 1	(I)Input 2	(O)Output 1	DMU	(I)Input 1	(I)Input 2	(O)Output 1
1	9.19680082	9.11250601	1	51	9.357032954	9.147920391	1
2	6.98329723	9.0759965	1	52	2.016895472	9.173779199	1
3	2.65870136	9.08328407	1	53	3.509031645	9.111827184	1
4	4.85869829	9.18288254	1	54	9.292785595	9.161303244	1
5	2.27595829	9.18945063	1	55	2.565717034	9.121923819	1
6	7.03352883	9.0980845	1	56	1.743224922	9.041879766	1
7	2.7886742	9.15050184	1	57	5.624698858	9.160226883	1
8	8.32154394	9.0806671	1	58	1.414046739	9.150767692	1
9	2.9669212	9.12536664	1	59	8.973385043	9.083885619	1
10	4.01680894	9.1067919	1	60	5.804010133	9.150058877	1
11	1.40635449	9.1508407	1	61	8.252179457	9.073432399	1
12	5.67889473	9.05590478	1	62	7.714140135	9.080894692	1
13	5.82390832	9.01941995	1	63	8.874414332	9.000604287	1
14	7.17462201	9.029073	1	64	8.674756711	9.122493386	1
15	3.53835347	9.03210469	1	65	1.37131667	9.141494461	1
16	6.15180033	9.137801	1	66	1.81317429	9.001828253	1
17	2.68653386	9.15927131	1	67	6.852949381	9.041589967	1
18	3.74581345	9.04024703	1	68	2.479890316	9.032429966	1
19	3.36755963	9.02784117	1	69	8.129091123	9.074929631	1
20	7.98751009	9.10534761	1	70	1.437994084	9.155841554	1
21	1.91280888	9.06108151	1	71	3.915752845	9.114873709	1
22	8.77461916	9.19876259	1	72	8.856856034	9.160930268	1
23	6.32857927	9.19635998	1	73	1.630149262	9.168182081	1
24	2.39676315	9.02627165	1	74	7.194408829	9.168589726	1
25	6.38003953	9.09336426	1	75	4.840963581	9.022984101	1
26	3.29606983	9.14479497	1	76	6.405731746	9.102304193	1
27	4.18525247	9.03810629	1	77	6.228921118	9.001056818	1
28	2.37231253	9.09168147	1	78	4.398406815	9.128207781	1
29	9.59395302	9.1591956	1	79	2.743484343	9.197692349	1
30	5.21240572	9.08848865	1	80	5.043862262	9.112212092	1
31	6.30068023	9.07120537	1	81	3.513704619	9.08084749	1
32	4.26110826	9.11334619	1	82	3.4119388	9.171196923	1
33	7.01767414	9.08958486	1	83	8.202261389	9.029952228	1
34	7.63272307	9.16098848	1	84	4.350558518	9.09745694	1
35	9.75235891	9.07984049	1	85	9.592884464	9.18566799	1
36	5.64960665	9.04964032	1	86	4.359503541	9.011221842	1
37	9.12660409	9.12099995	1	87	2.333047414	9.130261433	1
38	3.06159541	9.16591288	1	88	6.401022687	9.182136784	1
39	7.41947235	9.00588782	1	89	2.171614047	9.181148684	1
40	9.83295233	9.16495425	1	90	2.408242157	9.077059094	1
41	9.6657972	9.18062222	1	91	6.836334978	9.038342235	1
42	1.94449462	9.03788122	1	92	3.636684289	9.021456029	1
43	9.78991136	9.0969493	1	93	1.185269594	9.008671364	1
44	8.01940484	9.15696038	1	94	7.402972038	9.102754139	1
45	6.43134333	9.19607349	1	95	2.226871844	9.025583263	1
46	6.04890387	9.11221153	1	96	5.096362455	9.180494354	1
47	7.45146954	9.00791968	1	97	6.248479009	9.011465643	1
48	7.61883782	9.10084697	1	98	1.318957792	9.10031743	1
49	3.33725901	9.13346436	1	99	4.725853601	9.140195444	1
50	5.40127672	9.18419326	1	100	1.910540906	9.14138876	1

Table 7.2.4-3: Data set with big variations in input 1 and small variations in input 2.

Dimension	Quartiles	Mean Rank	z-value	double side p-value
	1 Quartile	59.6	6.06	<.0001
	2+3 Quartile	27.2		
Input 1	1 Quartile	37.4	-5.78	<.0001
	4Quartile	13.6		
	2+3 Quartile	50.4	-6.97	<.0001
	4Quartile	13.2		
	1 Quartile	40	-0.56	0.5755
	2+3 Quartile	37		
Input 2	1 Quartile	28.8	1.57	0.1164
	4Quartile	22.5		
	2+3 Quartile	40.7	1.48	0.1389
	4Quartile	32.7		

Table 7.2.4-4: Results of the MWU-Test for with small variations in input 2.

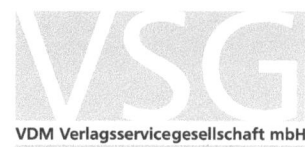

Die VDM Verlagsservicegesellschaft sucht für wissenschaftliche Verlage abgeschlossene und herausragende

Dissertationen, Habilitationen, Diplomarbeiten, Master Theses, Magisterarbeiten usw.

für die kostenlose Publikation als Fachbuch.

Sie verfügen über eine Arbeit, die hohen inhaltlichen und formalen Ansprüchen genügt, und haben Interesse an einer honorarvergüteten Publikation?

Dann senden Sie bitte erste Informationen über sich und Ihre Arbeit per Email an *info@vdm-vsg.de*.

Sie erhalten kurzfristig unser Feedback!

VDM Verlagsservicegesellschaft mbH
Dudweiler Landstr. 99   Telefon +49 681 3720 174
D - 66123 Saarbrücken   Fax   +49 681 3720 1749
www.vdm-vsg.de

Die VDM Verlagsservicegesellschaft mbH vertritt

 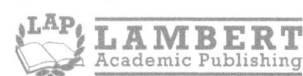 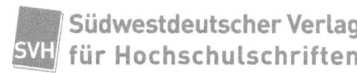

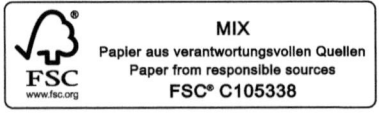

Printed by Books on Demand GmbH, Norderstedt / Germany